Talking Back to OCD

Talking Back to OCD

The Program That Helps Kids and Teens Say "No Way"— and Parents Say "Way to Go"

JOHN S. MARCH, MD
with Christine M. Benton

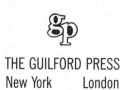

THE GUILFORD PRESS
New York   London

The information in this volume is not intended as a substitute for consultation with healthcare professionals. Each individual's health concerns should be evaluated by a qualified professional.

Many children and teenagers with OCD and their parents have generously and courageously shared their thoughts and feelings with me over the years, but to protect their privacy we have used only composites in this book. The descriptions and quotes accurately reflect the typical experiences of my patients and their families, but all names, ages, and other identifying details have been changed, as has the wording of their quotes.

Library of Congress Cataloging-in-Publication Data

March, John S., MD
    Talking back to OCD : the program that helps kids and teens say "no way"—and parents say "way to go" / by John S. March, with Christine M. Benton.
        p. cm.
    Includes bibliographical references and index.
    ISBN 978-1-59385-355-6 (pbk.: alk. paper)
    ISBN 978-1-59385-356-3 (hardcover: alk. paper)
    1. Obsessive–compulsive disorder in children—Popular works.   2. Obsessive–compulsive disorder in adolescence—Popular works.   I. Benton, Christine M.
II. Title.
    RJ506.O25M375 2007
    618.92'85227—dc22

                                                        2006024322

Contents

Preface

One in 200 young people suffers from obsessive–compulsive disorder (OCD). This means there are 3–4 youngsters with OCD in every average-size elementary school and up to 20–30 in every high school. Many don't know they have OCD—or, better said, they don't know what to call it. Of those who do, most don't have access to expert cognitive-behavioral therapy (CBT). Research tells us that CBT is the best treatment for OCD, far better than doing nothing and a lot better than medications. The purpose of this book is to bring CBT to kids and parents and so to help reduce the suffering of children and teenagers with OCD and their families.

Fifteen years ago, when I first began to figure out how to do CBT with kids, practicing clinicians routinely complained that children refused to comply with treatment, while parents complained that most clinicians didn't know how to use CBT to treat OCD in young people. The initial efforts to improve this situation in the OCD treatment program at Duke University Medical Center led to How I Ran OCD Off My Land©, a name given to our program by a young man who was one of our first treatment successes. In 1998, this treatment program was published in a book for therapists entitled *OCD in Children and Adolescents: A Cognitive-Behavioral Treatment Manual*, and it has since become the standard of care around the world for pediatric OCD.

In developing the first treatment manual, our goals were simple: (1) to encourage compliance by our young patients and their parents, (2) to create a program that would work in a wide variety of clinical settings, and (3) to facilitate the scientific evaluation of and improvements in OCD treatment. To speed adoption of CBT by the therapist community, my colleagues and I tried to incorporate the many "clinical pearls" that, in our experience, make CBT practical and effective for kids and teens with OCD. Unfortunately, there are still not enough therapists using CBT to treat all the young people with OCD who could benefit from it. At Duke we get e-mails every day from parents who are desperate to find a therapist who could use CBT with their child. Many parents bought our book for therapists and used it themselves or took it with them to their child's therapist with a request to switch to this effective treatment strategy. We wrote this book for you to use whether you have a therapist or not. After all, no one cares for a child more than his or her parents, and nobody knows OCD as well as the young person who has it. Who better to get on the same page in running OCD out of your life? You need an owner's guide to OCD, and this is it.

In writing this book, we tried to follow the same procedures used every day in the OCD treatment program at Duke University Medical Center. As with the book for therapists, each chapter has a specific set of goals that build on the preceding chapters. It is very important to read the whole book and then work through it chapter by chapter. In developing this program, my colleagues and I have seen and treated many hundreds of children and adolescents and have provided more than 4,000 hours of hands-on therapy for OCD. Along the way, we've made plenty of mistakes and taken lots of therapeutic detours, most of which you can avoid by following the program carefully. Children and families react differently to OCD, and OCD varies tremendously in its manifestations, so feel free to improvise when circumstances dictate.

While it has been my good fortune to participate in the development and dissemination of CBT for pediatric OCD, many others also deserve credit. Most of all, I owe a special debt of gratitude to the many patients and their families who have taught my colleagues and me so much about OCD in kids. With so much of mental health care still driven by ineffective relationship-oriented psychotherapies, it often seems that our patients and their parents are ahead of the field in their understanding of OCD as a neuropsychiatric disorder. Their thoughtful observations, cheerfulness in the face of OCD, and willingness to explore with us as we worked the kinks out of the treatment have been both professionally helpful and personally rewarding. Above all, the pleasure of watching a child's enthusiasm for successfully "bossing back OCD" increase as treatment proceeds drives my commitment to this work. I thank my patients and their families for the privilege of helping them.

This book builds on the work of many people. In the 1970s, when behavioral psychotherapy for OCD was still novel, Isaac Marks and his colleagues at the Institute for Psychiatry in London clearly demonstrated that exposure-based interventions worked for adults with OCD. Subsequently, gifted psychologists and psychiatrists—among them Lee Baer, Edna Foa, and John Greist—extended the reach of behavioral psychotherapy and systematized its application in adults. Our work is merely an extension of theirs. The National Institute of Mental Health group—Judith Rapoport, Henrietta Leonard, and Susan Swedo—readily shared their insights about pediatric OCD and encouraged the development of CBT for young persons with this disorder. Edna Foa and Martin Franklin have been inspiring and expert guides in helping to extend the benefits of CBT to children and adolescents. My colleague and coauthor on the first edition of the book for therapists, Karen Mulle, helped bring to life many of the clinical vignettes that informed this work.

Taken collectively, the work of these extraordinary clinician-researchers powerfully influenced my thinking; their friendship and generosity have been equally important to the success of this program.

As with the book for therapists, the able and patient support of Kitty Moore, Executive Editor at The Guilford Press, has been invaluable. Her wise counsel and honest desire to see a wider dissemination of scientific knowledge are primary causes for the publication of this text.

There is of course much more to life than academia, and my coauthor and I want to thank family and friends for their love and support, which make all other things, including the varied tasks of academic life, possible. I especially want to thank my colleagues at Duke University for their tireless efforts on behalf of mentally ill children, adolescents, and adults.

The whole edifice of medicine is based on a few researchers and their patients participating in clinical trials. Please visit *www.pcaad.org* to find out what we are up to in our current research projects. If you are working with a child and adolescent psychiatrist, please encourage your doctor to sign up to participate in the Child and Adolescent Psychiatry Trials Network (*www.captn.org*). As has been the case with cancer in young people, getting the practice community involved in research will give us the tools we need to improve the lives of mentally ill children.

Finally, as in most areas of psychiatry and psychology, controversy abounds. This book, while rich in information, will in some instances not do justice to the edge of the field, and the reader may not agree with everything we say. The errors of fact are ours; the controversies will eventually yield to good science. Our goal in producing this manual is to help children and adolescents with OCD lead more normal, happy, and productive lives. We hope we have achieved this goal.

JOHN S. MARCH

Introduction:
An Important Message for Parents

OBSESSIVE-COMPULSIVE DISORDER (OCD) is a brain illness. Kids and teenagers with OCD have mental "hiccups" (obsessions) that make them feel anxious or uncomfortable, and their illness tricks them into trying to eliminate that feeling by performing certain rituals over and over (compulsions). The obsessions that bother your son or daughter and the compulsions your child obeys to try to feel better don't seem to make much sense. So you and your child have probably tried hard to find a way to stop OCD. The trouble is, you've probably also found that sensible measures don't work too well against nonsensical OCD. If you're like most families, you probably feel confused and frustrated because you don't know where to turn.

That's where this book comes in. In Part II are eight steps that those ages 4 and up can use to get rid of the obsessions and compulsions that may be ruling your family's life. I devised this plan 15 years ago and have helped many hundreds of kids and teens use it to get rid of OCD and get on with their lives. Lots of other doctors use it, too, so we know it works. And now what we've been seeing in our offices has been confirmed by a large 5-year research study: This approach is the most effective way to get rid of mild to moderate OCD, and even kids who are bothered with more severe OCD do really well with this program. They might need lots of help from a therapist, might sometimes need to take medications as well, and might not get rid of obsessions and compulsions altogether. But any child or teen with OCD who uses this program stands an excellent chance of getting well enough to go on with school, friendships, sports, and the rest of normal life.

If this sounds good to you, read on.

What It Means to "Talk Back to OCD"

The program that we've found so successful in treating kids with OCD is based on cognitive-behavioral therapy (CBT), now considered to be the most successful general approach to eliminating OCD in both children and adults. In particular, the program is a type of exposure and response prevention (EX/RP) treatment. Put simply, it's a way of helping kids learn, very gradually, that if they resist the urge to perform the rituals that OCD demands, their obsessions and the anxiety or discomfort that comes with them will go away, little by little, over time.

We call this "talking back to OCD," because kids with this illness might feel as if they are being bossed around by OCD, forced to think about things they don't want to think about and then forced to complete certain actions to silence the thoughts and ease their discomfort. Our program gives them the confidence to boss OCD back. As they see that they can, in fact, shut OCD up, their confidence increases and they make more and more progress toward eliminating OCD from their lives.

If you've been trying to deal with OCD on your own for a while, you probably already know that "obeying" OCD only seems to make things worse. Maybe obsessions have been bothering your child more than ever, and it seems to take more and more hand washing, counting, arranging, or other rituals to make your son or daughter feel better. Using the tools we provide in this book will give you a proven way to turn OCD around.

How to Use This Book

My use of the kid-friendly term "talking back to OCD" to name this program is no accident. You may be surprised to know that your child will essentially be in charge of working his or her way toward eliminating OCD. We're talking to you parents right now because we know you're the ones who buy books like this. And you're the ones who are trying to find a way to help your child get rid of OCD. That's great. But in this program your child will be in charge and you'll play a supporting role rather than the lead. Here's a rundown of how it works:

Part I is essentially for parents, although some children and most adolescents would benefit from reading this part of the book as well. Read Part I first, to gain a working knowledge of what the illness called OCD is, what it looks like, what causes it, and how it can be treated effectively. Part I includes a lot of important concepts and principles on which the kids' program is based. Understand those and you'll have what you need to support your son or daughter in eliminating OCD.

Next, read through the program in Part II to get an understanding of what your child or teenager will be doing. Understanding the basic concepts and framework of the program will help you decide whether your son or daughter seems likely to be able to follow the eight steps and, if so, how much help he or she might need.

This book has been designed essentially to be used as a self-help manual, because I've found that kids with mild or moderate OCD and no other complicating illnesses can often follow the instructions for each step on their own. They still need their parents to be there to support, cheer, and provide help when asked, but many kids in middle school and up can essentially do the work independently.

If you have any doubt that your child can do this and that you too will be comfortable in the self-help mode, talk to a therapist who is willing to follow the program in our companion guide for therapists, *OCD in Children and Adolescents: A Cognitive-Behavioral Treatment Manual*, also published by The Guilford Press. (If you don't already have a therapist with experience in treating children with OCD, page 259 will help you find one.) The therapist should be able to help you figure out what will work best for your family—self-help, guided self-help (checking in with a therapist through regularly scheduled appointments), or just having the therapist "on call" for consultation as needed. I recommend that you consider having a therapist in the wings to help if needed, because just knowing a professional is there to back you up can boost your own confidence. And knowing who to call in advance means that you won't waste any time figuring out what to do if your child and you get stuck at some point in the program.

The instructions in Part II are adaptable. You can use them regardless of the level of help you plan to enlist and whatever your child's needs and abilities may be. The instructions for each step speak directly to your son or daughter. If your child is, say, age 10 or older, she can read and follow them on her own. (We've provided separate suggestions for teenagers in recognition that they are, and insist on being treated as, a different group from younger kids.) The kids' instructions for each step are followed by a section for parents (on the tabbed pages) that help you carry out your part. In these sections you'll find tips for providing the extra help that younger kids may need, clues to when to call in a therapist if your child gets stalled, and creative ideas for being the best cheerleader and coach you can be.

In a sense, you're getting two books in one: a child manual and a parent manual. Chapter 5, at the beginning of Part II, will help you figure out how to put them together in the best way for your family—whether you should sit down and talk about each step together before your child launches into the work, how often you should check in with each other, how you'll evaluate progress and know when to move to the next step, and so forth.

But first, once you've determined that this program might work for your child and family, you should introduce the book and the program to your son or daughter. If your child is old enough or sophisticated enough to grasp the material in Part I, by all means he or she should read it, too. If not, we've included lots of boxes that tell you how to pass on what you're reading to your child by talking about OCD in a brand-new way. This is a good way for you to lay the groundwork for your child's success with the eight steps in Part II.

Also critical to success is a mutual understanding of how long the program should take. Although progress is gradual, it's important not to take much longer than 4 months to complete the eight steps. If you stretch it out, your child won't gain confidence quickly enough, and progress may stall. (If you need more than 4 or 5 months, you almost certainly need the help of a therapist.) Move too fast, on the other hand, and the child may find the discomfort of OCD intolerable and want to give up. You and your child should be in agreement on this ahead of time so that you're not tempted to try to control the pace once the program begins. As we explain on page 5, it's important for your child to stay in charge, and that means no "nagging" from Mom or Dad to pick up the pace or slow it down. You shouldn't feel any need, anyway; the program teaches your child how to judge when it's time to move forward and provides plenty of incentive for doing so.

What to Tell Your Child about the Program

When you do present the program and the book to your child, tell your son or daughter that you've just read a good book by a doctor from Duke University who figured out how to treat OCD in young people, and it's given you a new way to think about OCD that you think may help your child get rid of OCD once and for all. Remind your child that all of you have been doing what you can without any success, and that it's no one's fault. You've all been doing your best, but OCD doesn't come with a manual that tells you how to make it go away: This book is the guide you've been looking for. Say that the program in this book is going to put your child, not OCD, back in charge. Following this program may mean that your child won't have to be bossed around by OCD anymore. And the whole thing will be in your child's control. You'll be there to help at all times, but your child will be the boss.

Say that you know your son or daughter can do it—and, of course, that you'll love your child no matter what.

A Whole New You . . . , or Why You Have to Put Your Child in Charge

Before you get started, it's important to be aware that this program requires a parental shift in attitude and behavior that may feel really unnatural. In fact, it may even feel like an abandonment of parental protectiveness and authority. Here's why it's not—why it's essential that you change how you've been approaching OCD so the program can work the way it's supposed to work.

First, the program's success depends on your backing off from helping with rituals, but in a very specific and controlled way. You probably know what I mean: Ben says he just can't go to school yet, because his socks aren't evened up and his shoes don't feel quite right. So you offer to help get it all straightened up and balanced so he can get to school on time. The job Ben has been assigned by OCD gets done, and he gets to the bus stop in the nick of time. Or Brooke gets more and more upset if she's not 100% sure that the dishes used to set the table for dinner are perfectly clean, so she asks you over and over about individual dishes and silverware, and you spend the predinner hour saying "Yes, honey, I washed the spoons. . . . Sure, Brooke, the dishwasher got nice and hot, and the plates are all as clean as they can get. . . . No, that's not a spot on your milk glass. . . . OK, I'll wash that one again."

If you've been trying to soothe your child's anxiety by going along with rituals like these, you already know that completing rituals stops your child's discomfort for the time being but that then the obsessions come galloping back. In fact, they come back stronger and more frequently than ever. So even though it feels only natural to do whatever you can to "make it all better," you have to learn how to stop helping your child with OCD rituals. They don't help your child feel better in the long run; they only make OCD grow. Surprisingly, it'll be your child who gives you permission to stop doing OCD's bidding. Right now all that's required is patience and kindness, plus taking the program outlined in this book to heart. We'll explain how this works in Part I, and throughout Part II we'll provide plenty of ways you can ease your child's discomfort without helping her give in to OCD's demands.

Second, the program works only when the person who talks back to OCD is the child who has the illness. Parental authority is second nature, every bit as much as parental protection, and putting your child in charge of "curing" his own illness may feel like letting a 7-year-old plan and cook his own meals. Naturally, you'll want to ensure that your child gets the most he can out of this program. But the way to do that is to let him set the pace, determine what works best, and do all the talking back to OCD. It's the only way his mind can internalize the fact that the discomfort accompanying obsessions isn't intolerable and that performing OCD rituals isn't the only way to make the obsessions go away. This is how EX/RP works. Hanging in there without performing a ritual reveals to your child that the discomfort doesn't get worse, as expected, but better. But that can happen only as long as the child is the one to say no to OCD and as long as, each time he resists OCD, he is successful. Your son or daughter has to be able to say "Yeah, this isn't fun, but to beat OCD I can stand to feel this crummy for this long." With that revelation cemented in his mind, your child gains increasing confidence to keep talking back to OCD. When you're in charge, your child will never truly believe that OCD can be controlled.

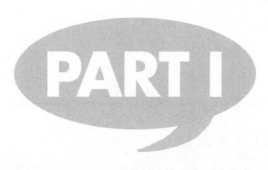

Up Close but Not So Personal

A NEW LOOK AT OCD FOR PARENTS (AND KIDS)

What Is OCD?

WHEN FAMILIES COME TO ME distraught over the fact that they haven't been able to get rid of a child's or teenager's OCD on their own, I start by telling them that OCD does not respond to sensible solutions because it is not an ordinary problem of daily life. Kids with OCD are normal kids up against a not-so-normal challenge. OCD is an illness, and, like any serious illness, it makes life harder for everyone in the family. The child or teenager feels miserable about not being able to get control over the "silly ideas" and "crazy behavior" of OCD. Parents worry about the future and feel guilty that they don't know how to help. Often everyone is frustrated with each other.

The trouble is that it can be difficult to view OCD as an illness in the brain. Kids with OCD are well aware that their obsessions and compulsions make no sense. That recognition makes them think it should be a simple matter to talk themselves out of listening to the obsessions or acting on the compulsions. Their parents, too, know their kids aren't "crazy," and so they try commonsense means to get rid of OCD. They may try reasoning with the child, cajoling, or even disciplining the child. Upset by the pain their child is feeling, they give her reassurance, comfort, and lots of affection. When none of this eliminates OCD, everyone in the family feels helpless and increasingly hopeless, and OCD thrives when the blame game gets going.

A shift in perspective works wonders. OCD is not about good or bad behavior. When you understand that OCD is a true brain illness, you realize that having it is not a matter of choice and resolving it is not a matter of willpower, though it does require good intentions. OCD is no more a matter of choice than is diabetes or asthma. And, as with diabetes and asthma, there are strategies for making OCD better, for living a normal life that is not constantly restricted by the illness. This view of OCD does, however, have its limits. Although diabetes or asthma often requires family members to adjust the way they think, feel, and act, these illnesses do not *cause* the child to think, feel, and act differently than before the disease struck. OCD does, and the typical family of a child with OCD can't help being frightened by these changes and feeling at a loss to deal with them.

This is where another perspective comes to the rescue, one that professionals helping kids with OCD have adopted almost universally. Think of having OCD as like having a bad case of mental hiccups—the term aptly assigned to OCD by Judith Rapoport in her groundbreaking book *The Boy Who Couldn't Stop Washing*. No matter how hard your child and you try to stop them, the embarrassing and senseless obsessions of OCD keep popping up, and your child keeps feeling as if he must perform certain repetitive actions in response. Like the hiccups, OCD may not seem so bad at first. But as time goes on, the hiccups get harder and harder to live with. If you had hiccups that not only refused to go away but got worse, it probably wouldn't be long before you felt as if you were trying to fit in breathing, speaking, eating, and every other function between hiccups. As you undoubtedly know, that's the way kids and families challenged by OCD often feel. You may feel like you're squeezing your ordinary lives in around the demands of OCD, wherever OCD will let you.

WHAT TO SAY TO YOUR CHILD ABOUT OCD

"OCD hiccups bugging you again?" Remembering that OCD is an illness—not some personal flaw, naughtiness, or craziness—and responding skillfully whenever you see that your child is being plagued by obsessions or compulsions will go a long way toward changing everyone's perspective about OCD.

Billy is a 9-year-old third grader who came to us with severe OCD. Billy's father had had OCD as a child and, as an adult, recognized it right away, so he brought Billy in for treatment. Nonetheless, Billy felt to blame for not being able to control OCD, saying angrily, "I can't make my mind do what I tell it." Once OCD was renamed as a hiccup in his brain, not something he was responsible for, Billy brightened up considerably, asking spontaneously, "OK, how do I make these stinking hiccups stop?"

The first step is to understand what OCD is and how it operates. With that knowledge as your foundation, your child and you will learn how to respond skillfully to obsessions and compulsions so that they get weaker and weaker and you all get your lives back.

OCD Is Everywhere

One of the most important things for all of you to know is that you're not alone. As is the case with other medical illnesses, such as diabetes and asthma, kids with OCD are all over the place. The latest statistics tell us that as many as 1 in every 200 children or teenagers has OCD today—about the same number of kids who have diabetes. That means that four or five kids with OCD are likely to be enrolled in any average-size elementary school. In a medium to large high school, there could be 20 students struggling with the challenges imposed by OCD. In adults, OCD is third among the most common forms of mental illness, almost three times more common than schizophrenia. Most of these adults had OCD as children, and back then they didn't have access to programs like this one. (If they had, maybe they would not be so troubled by OCD as adults.) In children and teens, OCD is also among the more common forms of mental illness, about a sixth as common as ADHD or depression, for example.

Knowing that your family is not alone in having to deal with OCD should make it easier for all of you to keep working together to help the child with OCD get better. You can help your child understand this by saying something like what appears in the sidebar.

Knowing your family isn't alone in this struggle helps for several reasons. First of all, there's comfort in numbers. A problem that affects hundreds of thousands of children in the United States alone can hardly be viewed as the exotic problem it may seem to be close up, in isolation. Throughout this book you'll meet many people who are sharing your challenges, and if that's not enough to ease your mind, a doctor who has seen many children with OCD will be able to assure you that you're in good company. Viewing OCD from this broad perspective may be just what the whole family needs to step back, take a deep breath, and begin the work of fighting back—together.

> **WHAT TO SAY TO YOUR CHILD ABOUT OCD**
>
> "Did you know that there are other kids around you at school who are struggling with OCD just like you? In fact, the student sitting next to you in class is about as likely to have OCD as diabetes. Four or five kids with OCD are likely to be enrolled in any average-size elementary school. In a medium to large high school, there could be 20 students dealing with OCD. Normal kids have diabetes; normal kids have OCD. You're just sick—temporarily. You're not so 'different' after all!"

Second, there's help in numbers. If OCD is so widespread, then there is a huge number of other people who can recommend strategies they have found successful, warn you of pitfalls they've stumbled into, and offer emotional support when you need it. Kids who are successfully fighting OCD characteristically demonstrate enormous courage and generosity in sharing their experiences to help others. A perfect example is the kids (and their parents) whose stories have enriched our understanding of how OCD works and how to beat it and whom you'll read about throughout this book. Your doctor or therapist should be able to refer you to local sources of ongoing support, and the Resources section in this book contains a list of organizations.

One of the cool things about going to the clinic was the chance to meet other teenagers with OCD and their parents. We'd sit in the waiting room and tell stories about what OCD was doing and how we'd found ways to beat it at its own game using the approaches we learned. Once Chad was really getting better, what was really neat was to listen to him telling other kids who were just getting started,

and weren't quite sure they wanted to buy into it, how great it was to be able to put OCD aside and get on with stuff he liked doing instead. Seeing the other kids brighten up really made him feel good about himself and what we were doing.
                                        —Maggie, mother of 14-year-old Chad

Third, where the numbers go, the research follows. Scientists today know more about OCD in kids than about just about any other mental problem except attention-deficit/hyperactivity disorder (ADHD). That's due in part to the ability and willingness of kids with OCD to describe their experiences and also participate in research projects. We've found in our research, in fact, that kids and parents are often smarter and more informed about OCD than mental health professionals are, and this has led to dramatic strides in advocating for better treatments. But recognition of the large number of kids and adults harmed by OCD has led to studies at Duke University, the University of Pennsylvania, and other research centers around the world. We now have a wealth of new information about what causes OCD (see Chapter 3), and—the best news of all—we have made huge strides in treating it (see Chapter 4). So much so, in fact, that we can realistically hope to reduce the rates of OCD significantly among children and adults in the not too distant future.

OCD Is Sneaky

Probably the greatest benefit of realizing you're not alone with OCD is that it gets OCD out in the open as an illness. OCD is not a part of who your child is, nor did you do anything to cause it. Once OCD is revealed as an illness, it becomes obvious that it's not the child's or parents' fault, any more than diabetes would be someone's fault. It is your responsibility to address OCD skillfully, however. Relieving themselves of guilt makes it much easier for most families to move from what hasn't worked to what does work. A survey of 5,000 high school students done in the late 1980s found 18 students who had OCD, but *none of them had been identified as having OCD, including the 4 who were seeing a psychiatrist or psychologist.* OCD is a bit more likely to be diagnosed these days, but nowhere near often enough, in part because many kids don't want to tell anyone they have a problem. This means that the 1-in-200 figure we quoted earlier may be just the tip of the iceberg, with OCD being even more common than we imagined. One scientist, in fact, called OCD a "hidden epidemic" because so few young people who have OCD are identified as having it and even fewer receive appropriate treatment.

It's not surprising that OCD often remains hidden, because the disturbing thoughts, pictures, or urges that we call *obsessions* and that pop up in the mind for no apparent reason might make an odd kind of sense to the child at first. Children have incredible powers of imagination, and fantasizing is a critical tool they use to understand and adapt to a large and sometimes scary world. In addition, lots of behaviors that are out of whack in OCD are pretty normal in other contexts: washing hands before dinner, insisting on a nightly bedtime story, arranging dolls, or, for teens, spending a fair amount of time getting dressed and grooming. It might be difficult at the start for a child to see the difference between obsessing about getting germs in the bathroom that she fears she will pass on to her mother and worrying about the fact that the bathroom at school really can be disgustingly dirty. Washing her hands a lot to get rid of germs when it really isn't necessary—the repetitive actions we call

WHAT TO SAY TO YOUR CHILD ABOUT OCD

"OCD tries to trick you into thinking that what it wants you to do makes sense. You know it doesn't, but it can feel pretty real, especially when you're in the middle of it. Pretty soon you're going to find out that nothing about OCD is real except that it bugs you and that if you don't do what OCD says, it'll leave you alone."

compulsions—might not seem much different from the ordinary routine of washing your hands before dinner. After all, many people do wash before dinner, so why should she believe, at least at first, that washing her hands isn't a sensible thing to do?

> *OCD made me wash my hands whenever I would touch something that felt dirty or germy. At the beginning, I just thought OCD was something I had to do to keep safe because my little brother had leukemia and we all had to wash our hands a lot, but I realized real fast that it was more than what other kids did. Even my little brother didn't worry or wash his hands as much as I did.*
>
> —*Susie, age 11*

At the beginning, many children might in fact view the rituals or compulsions as offering pretty helpful advice and warnings. When children perform rituals, the frightening or disturbing feelings that accompany their obsessions usually go away for a little while. OCD can be trusted, the child thinks. But wait. As time goes on, the young girl just described felt like she had to wash her hands not 5 or even 10 times a day but 20, then 30, then 50. Or she felt compelled to wash her hands not just after going to the bathroom but after touching any other person, eating food, or riding in a car. Before she and her family knew what had hit them, OCD was in control of the child's waking hours, and everyone felt worse and worse—even though by that time Susie had no doubt that OCD made no sense at all.

In short, OCD fools kids into thinking the whole scheme makes sense—after all, washing one's hands *is* the right thing to do to rid them of germs. It says so on TV. Even when kids know that OCD makes no sense, which is true of most kids most of the time, this realization only makes them keep silent for fear of being labeled "crazy." Or they have tried so valiantly yet unsuccessfully to bounce OCD out of their brains that they feel hopeless, stuck with OCD forever. Or the intrusive thoughts that torment them feel shameful and fill them with guilt; they don't dare admit to being as "bad" as their thoughts tell them they are. The result in all cases is that it might take parents months, even a year or two, to figure out that they have a

> **WHAT TO SAY TO YOUR CHILD ABOUT OCD**

"Just because OCD makes you feel bad—and sometimes feel bad about yourself—doesn't mean you *are* bad. The thoughts that make you feel crummy are coming from OCD. They're not part of who you are—a good, smart, neat kid who just happens to have OCD."

child who needs help. (Adults with OCD have the same reactions. Those who first notice OCD in their 20s often don't ask for help for 8 or more years!)

When it started, I had this thought that if I looked at a guy's butt, it meant I wanted to have sex with him, so I tried hard not to look. It didn't take long before the other kids asked me why I was always looking at the floor or staring off somewhere else. Since I was too embarrassed to tell the truth, I told them I was shy or that the sun or lights bothered me. Eventually, no one asked anymore. They just ignored me. Before I found out that this was OCD, I lost all my friends. I felt so alone.

—Anna, age 13

The messages that are sent by the illness called OCD aren't true, just as many other thoughts that pop up in your mind every day aren't true. But unlike these other brain moments, OCD thoughts won't go away by themselves. That's why we call them brain "hiccups." They hang around and around and around, provoking unpleasant feelings and rituals as the child desperately tries to get back in control. For example, a typical OCD thought tells a child that her mother will get sick if she doesn't wash her hands 50 times each day, with the consequence that the child feels terrible—frightened, guilty, forlorn—even as she washes her hands over and over, knowing it makes no sense. Mom is just fine. But OCD is never satisfied. Like an ogre with a great big hungry mouth, it never gets enough to eat. The child who faithfully fulfills OCD's demands today is rewarded tomorrow with even tougher tasks to complete. *In our experience with many hundreds of kids with OCD, it is painfully clear that nobody hates OCD more than the young men or women who have it.* OCD is never on their side, and the fact that they are capable of realizing that gives children a huge boost toward being able to boot OCD out of mind once and for all.

OCD Doesn't Belong Here

Most children—and their parents—fully understand that what OCD is telling them is untrue and unfair. But how do they reconcile that fact with the fact that OCD can look for all the world like bad behavior? Many families plagued by OCD have great difficulty separating the disorder from the child victimized by it. This is why some parents discipline their children for not obeying their orders to "just stop it." It's why some children give up their lives to their compulsions in a short-term bargain to halt the obsessions that ultimately seem so goofy. But if we look at the origins of the words "obsession" and "compulsion," it's easy to see that OCD can and should be viewed as something outside the child's personality that has invaded the child's life territory. "Obsession" comes from the Latin word *obsidere*, which means "to besiege," and "compulsion" comes from the Latin *compellere*, which means "to compel." What force is performing these actions? What is waging a siege against the child with OCD? What is compelling the child to perform senseless rituals over and over, day after day? Certainly not the child. It's the brain blips we call OCD.

> *Of course I know better than anybody that OCD is weird. I'm the one that has it. But it isn't always so easy. I mean it's easy here with my doctor, who understands that it isn't me and helps me understand that too. But when I'm alone and OCD is a hurricane and I'm doing the rituals and the thoughts keep pounding, sometimes I'm not so sure what's real anymore. I'm not crazy, but OCD sure drove me crazy before I learned how to keep it under control.*
>
> *—Tom, age 17*

OCD Is Not Insanity

How can we be so sure that OCD and not the child is playing this tune? Because children with OCD know that the obsessions in OCD make no sense and that the rituals are excessive and out of proportion to anything ordinary. This capacity is what we call *insight*, and it is something of a double-edged sword.

On the positive side, insight helps kids (and you, their parents) grasp the distinction between their illness and their personality. It's as if there's a supervisor in the brain that observes the obsessions and compulsions and recognizes that something is off. That supervisor could be thought of as the child himself or his personality. The OCD symptoms are something that can be separated out, like a stubbed toe or athlete's foot. The fact that the child already knows the obsessions and compulsions don't make sense and wants to get rid of them makes OCD easier to treat than illnesses such as schizophrenia, in which the person can't separate reality from delusions or hallucinations.

On the negative side, because they know full well that it makes no sense to keep on performing rituals, kids with OCD are often pretty tough on themselves for not being able to get rid of OCD just

WHAT TO SAY TO YOUR CHILD ABOUT OCD

"OCD is like athlete's foot. You know it's there—it itches and you scratch—*and* you know it's separate from the rest of you. That's going to make it a lot easier to get rid of."

by trying harder. It takes specific skills, not just seeing that OCD is not him, for your child to become his own boss again, which is why we developed this program and wrote this book.

I used to hate myself because of OCD. For years, I told myself that I was dumb because I kept doing praying rituals even though I knew that God would never want me to feel bad or do OCD. It wasn't until I recognized that OCD is just a disease and not me that I began to feel better and really not until I got a handle on OCD that I started to feel good about myself again.

—Adam, age 16

Although most young people are quite insightful about OCD being a mental hiccup different from their usual thoughts and feelings, insight can disappear or lessen during an attack of OCD. This is especially true in little kids. It is hard to keep it all straight when OCD is hollering loudly, especially before the child understands how to keep his distance from OCD. More commonly, insight seems to disappear (it really doesn't) when a child feels that he's being asked the impossible, namely to resist his rituals when he can't, and so must insist that they are necessary even when he knows that the opposite is true.

How you talk to a child or teen with OCD makes a huge difference in how insightful the young person may appear. Talk about OCD as it is—a plague on the child's planet—and insight sharpens; criticize or identify OCD with the person who has it, and insight often seems to go away as the child understandably becomes defensive. Very young children often haven't yet figured out all the ways to distinguish what is true from merely thinking that something is true, so they sometimes have a bit more trouble seeing OCD for what it is: disturbing nonsense. For these reasons, children and adolescents can be diagnosed with OCD without being so sure that their obsessions and compulsions are unreal. Remember, though, that it is very rare for the child or teenager with OCD not to know that obsessions are senseless and rituals excessive.

I didn't like it, having to touch my ear to keep Mommy from getting sick, but I had to 'cause I love her. She's my Mommy.

—Angela, age 4½

In my house, we always wash our hands before dinner, so it was hard at first to know what was normal and what was OCD.

—Joseph, age 15

My mom's a neat freak. So am I. But arranging and rearranging my clothes for hours—that's OCD, not being neat.

—Ally, age 12

In fact, insight is one of the distinctions in the diagnostic criteria for OCD in adults and OCD in children. To be diagnosed with OCD, adults *have to* understand that their obsessions are senseless, silly, irrational, illogical, and unreal, because adults are expected to have the mental maturity to make such distinctions. We don't require this of children, but it is generally true anyway.

If having OCD doesn't mean you're crazy, how do mental health professionals view it? OCD can be classified in a number of different ways. If you view mental illnesses as falling under various categories, the way a family tree is often drawn, at the top of the diagram OCD would be considered a medical disorder, as a disease of the mind that arises in the brain. "Disorder" means that OCD has been identified and defined in a way that all doctors who are trying to diagnose it will be able to agree on what they are talking about. Under the disorder category, OCD is currently put into the group called "anxiety disorders." Anxiety is worry that seems out of proportion and not very well connected to the situation facing the person. Though anxiety disorders are the most common mental disorders, many people don't take them as seriously as other types of mental illness, perhaps because they usually don't seem as severe as, say, bipolar disorder or as disruptive as ADHD. Finally, because many people with OCD don't really feel anxious during an OCD attack, and because some don't even have OCD thoughts, just urges or nagging feelings, we believe, as do many OCD researchers, that OCD belongs in its own category, along with the tic disorders, trichotillomania (compulsive hair pulling), and perhaps body dysmorphic disorder (obsessions about physical appearance).

Although, as just mentioned, not everyone who has OCD is aware of feeling fear or worry connected with obsessions, many children who have OCD perform their compulsions out of fear that failing to do so will bring on some terrible consequence, such as illness or death, either to the child or to someone else. And when they act on fearful thoughts and feelings by doing rituals, they are responding via a very primitive automatic mechanism in the brain. Fear, which is located in widely distributed emotion regulation centers, is one of the brain's most fundamental survival tools, and the specific obsessions and compulsions of OCD are "hardwired" in the brain. Two particular parts of the brain that have been implicated in OCD are the caudate nucleus, which controls the stop signal for habitual behaviors, and the orbital-frontal cortex (located right behind the eye), which controls complex emotions such as worry about harming others, guilt, and disgust.

When we say that OCD is a brain hiccup, we mean that we now know that OCD hijacks these brain centers. For example, when danger arises, certain brain structures sound a loud alarm and bring enough discomfort that the person will take immediate action to evade the danger and cut off the unpleasant sensations. After all, if someone sick sneezes on you, it makes sense to feel disgusted and to want to wash up right away. Responding this way seems hardly insane when viewed as a natural response dictated by the brain. The problem with OCD, of course, is that the

WHAT TO SAY TO YOUR CHILD ABOUT OCD

"OCD is like a stop signal in your brain that isn't working quite right. When it *should* get flipped to red so your brain stops worrying about something that OCD wants you to worry about, your brain gets stuck on green, and bingo—you're off to the OCD races. So what can we do about it? Let's fix the switch! That's what we're going to do with this book."

brain generates obsessions that trigger the unpleasant feelings and rituals even when there is no reason to be concerned. It is as though the brain registers a five-alarm fire when there isn't any smoke, and even when it knows better, it keeps the fire hoses spraying water. Because this is an automatic or habitual behavioral response, the person with OCD experiences it as something that happens to him. On the other hand, once OCD is recognized as OCD and the person learns more skillful ways to deal with it, giving in to OCD can change to active coping, which feels much better even though OCD still is firing off false messages.

> *I used to think I was the only one who was nuts until I heard how common OCD was and how it was just an illness. My therapist treats me like a real person, not some wacko. It took a while, but I finally told him all of it, even the really embarrassing parts. After five years of this *#$&*^, wow, what a relief!*
>
> —Sam, age 13

OCD Is a Neuropsychiatric Illness

The big question, then, is why those obsessions keep interrupting the child's normal thought process. In the field of health care, OCD is considered a neuropsychiatric illness—*neuro* because OCD is thought to originate in the brain and *psychiatric* because it affects thoughts, feelings, and behavior. That means it is biological, not caused by stress in the child's environment or by how you are raising your child. There isn't any secret lurking around in there that has to be uncovered. Something in your family isn't causing OCD. OCD is just what it is, OCD. That doesn't mean that things that happen can't trigger OCD or make it worse. Sometimes OCD begins right after a distressing event, such as a death or divorce or moving to a new town. Contamination fears often start with being sick. Just as often OCD comes out of the blue, kind of like the weather. OCD just happens. Because difficult things happen to lots of kids, it is often hard to know whether something stressful made OCD turn up. On the other hand, we can be sure that stress makes OCD more difficult to resist, so part of what we'll talk about later is how to reduce and manage stress, not because it causes OCD but because it is harder to successfully resist OCD if you're stressed out.

We'll go into what we know about the neurobiological causes of OCD in much more depth in Chapter 3. For now, a good way to understand what happens in the mind of a child is to view obsessions and compulsions as Judith Rapoport did, as hiccups coming from the brain. The mechanisms in the brain that should keep normal thought processes moving along without getting stuck malfunction in people with OCD, and the thoughts that would normally be tossed out as illogical or unimportant keep nagging at the child with OCD.

Thanks to enormous advances in brain imaging technology, we now know a lot about which circuits in the brain are associated with OCD. At one point late in the 20th century, researchers thought the problem lay solely with the neurochemical messenger serotonin, because experiments with medications showed that the selective serotonin reuptake inhibitors (SSRIs; see Chapter 4) helped people with OCD. Medications do help people with OCD, and for some people they are an important part

WHAT TO SAY TO YOUR CHILD ABOUT OCD

"Let's say you have a light switch that is stuck in the on position. Once you fix whatever is wrong with it, not only does the light go off and on like it should, but the light switch works like brand new. That's what can happen in your brain: You find a way to respond skillfully to OCD, and before you know it, that OCD switch doesn't get stuck 'on' at all."

of treatment. But the most amazing revelation is exactly what makes the program in this book so effective: that changing their relationship to OCD without medication can make children's brain circuits stop hiccupping, which means the obsessions that are making them so miserable miraculously cease, making rituals unnecessary.

Let's say it again. OCD is a brain illness. By taking control of how they respond to OCD, kids can change their brains so that OCD largely goes away, to be replaced by normal brain responses and normal behaviors.

So how does a child go about changing her relationship with OCD? By understanding and using everything we've talked about in this chapter so far:

- OCD is a mental hiccup that can't be trusted.
- It's like athlete's foot—an annoyance that can be eliminated, and not an innate, permanent part of the child.
- Children with OCD are not "crazy" but, to the contrary, typically are quite insightful and, incidentally, tend to be of average or greater intelligence.
- OCD originates in the brain rather than being caused by—and blamed on— the parents or some other facet of the child's upbringing.

These are all integral parts of the program we teach in this book. Because the program shows children how to use their minds to change their attitudes toward OCD and thus their day-to-day ways of coping with it, this program is called a form of *cognitive-behavioral therapy*. For children with mild to moderate OCD and, in some cases, even severe OCD (defined in Chapter 2), it can be even more effective than medication.

OCD Is an Impostor

This brings us to an important point that needs to be underscored for both parents and children if the child is to succeed in beating OCD. So far we have been describing OCD as an interloper with anything but good intentions. Closer to the truth is that OCD resembles those moustache-twirling villains from historic melodramas and more recent cartoons.

Everything I know, except how to beat OCD, I learned from The Simpsons. *How to whale on OCD, I learned from Dr. March. For OCD, he's a lot better than TV.*
                                                              —*Charles, age 12*

OCD that's been around for a while has a way of demeaning and demoralizing the child it torments. One form its treachery takes is to convince the child that he has a major flaw: "I must be really stupid, or I wouldn't keep having these thoughts and I wouldn't make my parents so miserable." That's just the illusion that this man-behind-the-curtain-posing-as-the-great-and-powerful-Oz wants everyone to buy.

The most effective way we know for both children and their parents to keep up their spirits while learning how to boss back OCD is to laugh gently at it while doing the opposite of what OCD wants. As we'll describe in Part II, some kids like to give OCD a humorous nickname to remind them that OCD is not a gigantic monster under the bed. Older kids can just keep reminding themselves that anything that wastes time repeating itself like this can't be all that fearsome—or nearly as smart as they are.

You know when I first knew that it was going to be OK? When my therapist asked me whether I wanted to give OCD a funny name or just wanted to call it OCD. Just asking the question made me smile inside. No one had ever talked to me about OCD like I was a real person before. Now we all do it, even my friends.
                                                              —*Sheila, age 14*

OCD Is Progressive—and It Can Be Reversed

If you're not yet convinced that OCD is conquerable, the best news for you is that OCD's most difficult feature is what makes it reversible. That is, although performing compulsions only makes OCD demand more and more from the child, gradually learning to resist the same compulsions has the opposite effect. If you don't play with OCD, it gets bored and goes away, *but only if you don't play with it.* Here's what happens before kids learn, through programs like the one in this book, to resist their compulsions:

Over long periods of time, research tells us that OCD has a tendency to get progressively worse or, at least, not to get much better. Most people with OCD recognize that obsessions are nonsensical and that compulsions are inappropriate and so resist them at least some of the time. After all, the person with OCD doesn't like doing these things and typically tries to stop giving in to OCD. Unfortunately, without the help offered in this program, failing at resisting is the rule rather than the exception, because OCD isn't easy to figure out without help. Otherwise, there wouldn't be any OCD. Take a teenage girl with germ fears and washing rituals. When she tries and fails to stop washing, her failure is likely to make her feel even more anxious, which then leads OCD to *confirm* that she has to give in to her compulsions. Giving in to OCD makes her feel helpless and ashamed, which only increases her anxiety, and the cycle continues. This doesn't mean the child with OCD is at fault for the disorder's progression, only that unwittingly playing into OCD's hands is part of the nature of the illness. To beat OCD, the child has to *win every time*, or the brain hiccups won't stop—it's not fair, but that's how it is. We'll show you how to do that step by step later in this book.

Occasionally, kids who don't learn to rein in OCD by getting effective treatment of a type that's been tested and proven in research studies find that "thinking about OCD" goes into overdrive and makes things worse. They start to have obsessive worries about whether their obsessions are true, a process we call doubting. The basic pattern seen in doubting is asking over and over "Is it OCD?" For example, a teenager with worries about whether he has "sinned" because of a "bad thought" may begin to doubt whether CBT is a good medical treatment or is "in league with the devil." When doubting happens, the program used in this book to teach kids how to think correctly about OCD becomes especially important.

Another consequence of untreated and worsening OCD in kids is that everyone in the family starts to try to help, usually to no good effect despite very good intentions. Parents, brothers, and sisters may end up participating in the rituals of the child with OCD or trying to prevent situations that they know trigger obsessions. Of course they're trying to help, but they're only making things worse. They're sending the message that compulsions actually do relieve obsessions, thus giving the OCD the go-ahead to make the child keep performing those rituals. Naturally, this means more and more of everyone's time will be taken up by OCD.

Fortunately, this trend can be turned around. Kids who succeed with the program in this book find that their obsessions stop soon after their rituals stop. These changes in the course of the disorder are borne out by brain imaging scans that show affected portions of the brain beginning to return to normal as treatment succeeds.

What to Expect from OCD

The course (how a mental disorder plays out over time) of OCD isn't entirely predictable, but we do know several things about it. First, without effective treatment, OCD tends to be a chronic mental disorder. That is, it lasts a long time and pretty much won't go away on its own, although it may wax and wane. That's the bad news. The good news is that the outcome of treatment is good to very good for most children who are able to get expert help in learning how to be the boss of OCD. Once it is gone, they can resume their normal lives, growing up just like other kids.

OCD varies widely in severity. Some kids have very mild OCD that stays mild, and they never seek help for it. (This is called "subclinical OCD"—OCD not severe

WHAT TO SAY TO YOUR CHILD ABOUT OCD

A few reminders for kids about what OCD *isn't*:

• *It's not "insanity."* "You're not crazy, even though it may feel like your obsessions are driving you crazy. OCD doesn't rob you of your power to think, and just because weird thoughts, images, or urges pop up in your brain doesn't mean you want to or will carry them out. You know your obsessions don't make sense, and that gives you a lot of power to run them out of your life. This book will help you do that. As Susie says: 'It's just my brain, hiccupping OCD, not me.' "

• *It's not just a few little habits.* "A lot of kids like you feel ashamed of their 'crazy' thoughts and rituals and so don't want to admit how big a problem OCD is causing them. But the fact that it's causing big trouble is one of the things that makes it OCD. OCD is not just a bunch of weird little habits. People generally develop habits for understandable reasons. Some people check their pockets several times to make sure their car keys are there because they have a history of misplacing them. Some people keep smoking even though they know it's bad for them because the nicotine in cigarettes is physically addictive, making it hard to quit. Other people bite their fingernails, but doing so doesn't keep them from doing what they do during a normal day or make them feel really bad. Baseball players spit and scratch or wear the same pair of lucky socks. OCD is different; it makes no sense, and it causes big-time trouble—there's nothing good about it. You aren't addicted to OCD, and OCD isn't a simple habit that you could quit or change if you only wanted to. OCD is an illness, and you deserve the chance to be rid of it."

• *OCD is not a sign that you're "bad."* "Some kids' obsessions are about hurting someone or saying or doing something harmful or inappropriate. One girl named Amy had the urge to stab her best friend with a fork, but only at her house. Because her friend, Taylor, didn't know that Amy had OCD, this caused a lot of trouble in their friendship as Amy stopped asking Taylor over to her house. This kind of thing does not mean you are in any way a bad person. Though very troubling, these obsessions make no more sense than any others and have nothing to do with who you really are. Once Amy told Taylor what was going on, Taylor was able to help Amy turn the tables on OCD using the tools presented in this program."

• *It's not your parents' fault.* "Although you might find the idea that OCD is our fault pretty attractive when we're acting particularly, well, parental, the truth is that scientists know OCD is not our fault any more than it's yours. We all need to learn how to react to OCD in a way that will get rid of it. No one in our family is to blame for OCD, and we're not going to listen to anyone, even a doctor, who says it is."

• *You're not brain damaged.* "Sure, some brain circuits are going off when they're not supposed to or, more to the point, they won't stop going off even though you want them to. Still, most things in your brain work just fine, and even the circuits in OCD can return to normal given the right treatment. More important, the things that make you whole as a person are fine. You are not OCD any more than having diabetes would mean that you as a person are diabetes. After all, millions of years of evolution came up with you, uniquely you, and we think you're pretty wonderful and worthy of deep respect from yourself, your family and friends, and your doctors."

enough to seek a doctor's attention.) In those cases the only way a doctor might recognize the problem may be in the course of seeing the child for something related to OCD. Sometimes the question of OCD pops up in the process of checking out a different medical problem. Kids who compulsively wash their hands out of fear of germs, for example, sometimes develop a hand rash related to washing, and the doctor may discover the compulsion when the child's mother makes an appointment to have the rash checked out. In most kids, OCD waxes and wanes—like the phases of the moon, only not as predictably. Sometimes symptoms seem to get better and sometimes they seem to get worse; usually they don't disappear altogether. A bit like the weather, attacks of OCD often come in bursts, usually for no particular reason, though significant stress, such as the start of school, can be expected to worsen symptoms in a lot of kids, simply because it makes it harder to resist OCD.

The outcome of OCD for any individual child depends on many factors, but, again, central among them is whether or not expert treatment is provided. Without expert treatment, a third to half of all children who have OCD likely would still have OCD, and often related problems, such as depression, as adults. In one follow-up study, 54 kids and teens diagnosed with OCD at the National Institute of Mental Health were looked at again 2–7 years later, and 43% of them could still be diagnosed with OCD. Only 11% had no OCD symptoms at all. Fortunately, this study was done many years ago, and, given expert treatment, kids can expect to do much better than this now (as our recent study has shown), but it is a warning that learning how to triumph over OCD is not optional. Without treatment, OCD will probably hang around for a long time.

Does everyone respond to treatment? Unfortunately, the answer is no, but most do. In our clinic, over 80% of patients eventually have no OCD symptoms that anyone else can see. Of those who still have bothersome symptoms that get in the way of daily living, most are considerably improved. For example, a boy or girl who was always late for school because of time-consuming bathroom rituals may still have some remaining rituals but isn't late anymore. How successful treatment will be depends on a number of factors, though getting expert cognitive-behavioral therapy (CBT) is the major factor that will improve the possibility of success. Having other disorders (such as depression) seems to make for a rougher road in adults, and the same is probably true for kids, but this just means that more treatments than just treatment for OCD will be required, and it may mean that it will also take a little longer to get well. And though family problems don't seem to cause OCD, one scientist found that a calm, supportive family atmosphere, which we help to set up at the beginning of treatment, may help a child with OCD get the most out of treatment.

Nine-year-old Hector came to treatment after struggling for 2 years with the need to get things arranged "just so" to keep something bad from happening. For example, he'd spend hours making sure that his socks were pulled up evenly, worrying that his mother would have a heart attack and die if he didn't do it. Although

Hector knew this was "nuts," he still felt responsible and so could not stop doing the rituals. With the assistance of his therapist "coach," Hector came to know OCD as OCD, namely as a neurobehavioral illness, not as something wrong with him as a person. With this beginning, Hector learned about OCD and how to talk to himself about OCD; his parents learned the same thing. With himself in control of the pace and using the skills he'd learned, Hector then went on to turn the tables on OCD by refusing to do OCD's rituals. Within 10 weeks, OCD was gone. That was 8 years ago, and, although OCD has tried several times to make a comeback, Hector, using the skills he learned and used effectively, never let OCD get a foothold. He's been well ever since and will start college next year.

2

What Does OCD Look Like?

THE SHORT ANSWER TO THIS QUESTION is that it depends on whether you're looking at OCD from inside or outside. If you were Andrew's mother or father, this is what you'd see:

Andrew came down for breakfast as he did on any school day morning and sat in his usual place at the kitchen table. His mother put a bowl of his favorite cereal in front of him, got the milk out of the fridge, and poured him a glass of juice. Then she turned back to the counter, where she was making out a list of chores for the kids to do after school while she was at work.

A few minutes later she realized she wasn't hearing any sounds of her son eating his breakfast. When she turned around to look, she saw Andrew sitting stock still, his chair pushed out from the table, his hands held stiffly against his body, a look of dread on his face.

"Honey, what's wrong?" she asked.

"I can't eat that," Andrew said in a voice that was clearly on the edge of tears.

"Why not?"

"It's dirty."

"*Nothing* on that table is dirty, Andrew. I spent five minutes making sure it was spotless before you even came down here! Now eat your breakfast before the bus gets here."

Here's what the same incident looked like to Andrew:

Andrew trotted down the stairs to the kitchen, carefully avoiding touching the banisters with his hands or brushing against them by staying right in

25

the middle of the steps. The first thing he saw when he got to the table was that his mother had put out a different spoon from the "dirty" silverware, not his special "clean" spoon. He froze for a second, feeling like some inner alarm system had been tripped. Why the new spoon? How could he be sure it was clean if it hadn't just come out of the dishwasher? Cautiously he pulled out his chair, holding his shirtsleeve over his hand to avoid direct contact, and sat down. As his mom brought out the milk and poured his juice, he noticed his napkin was on the right side of his bowl, not the left. And what was that little speck on the edge of his bowl? That juice glass didn't look as clean as it usually was when it came out of the dishwasher. Had his mom accidentally given him a glass that his sister had already used and just rinsed out? Maybe he better take a good look at the cereal. Was the milk fresh? He should probably just look at the expiration date on the carton, but then he'd have to get up, because it was on the other side of the carton from him and he didn't want to touch it until he was sure it was still OK. If he got up, his mom would notice and give him that look. . . .

If this scene played out, what Andrew's mom would see next would be her son tearfully asking her to get his regular spoon, clean the table again, give him a fresh bowl of cereal while he watched it being served, tell him the expiration date on the milk, and take a clean glass out of the dishwasher to pour him a new glass of juice. What Andrew would see would be the sheer impossibility of eating this breakfast as it was. He'd feel his mind reeling with the need to see with his own eyes the cleaning of everything on the table. At the same time, he'd feel ashamed, anxious, and a little afraid that his mother would yell at him, because going through this routine would mean he'd miss the bus and she'd have to drive him to school, which would make *her* late for work. But that would still be better than everyone dying from some strange illness that was his fault.

To get OCD out of Andrew's life (and out of your house), it's essential that both parents and child learn to see OCD through the same eyes. That can be a tall order, because obsessions (and even some compulsions) go on inside the child's head, and parents can't see in. All they can usually observe are OCD's effects on the child's outward behavior. And in many cases the visible outward behavior won't be entirely revealing. Many kids are ashamed of or embarrassed about the rituals that OCD makes them perform, and so they do their best to hide them. (In some cases, even people who see the child often, such as teachers, don't know a child has OCD because he has become so adept at hiding it—although this is possible only with certain types of obsessions and compulsions.) Also, rituals often change and become more complex and elaborate over time, making it hard for parents to see any connection between a particular compulsion and the obsession that OCD says the ritual will relieve. (Would you guess, when you repeatedly find your daughter's schoolbooks in the oven after she comes home from school, that she is trying to cleanse them of the "germs" OCD told her they'd picked up during the day?)

Depending on their age and the nature of the obsessions and compulsions, some kids can help their parents understand by explaining how they feel when OCD butts into their lives. But others can't say much more to explain why they feel compelled to count things or scrub their hands than "I just have to." Naturally this is frustrating for Mom and Dad—and sometimes sounds awfully similar to a child's explanation for wanting to stay up past bedtime or bypass some other rule: "I know it's late, but I just *have* to talk to Jenny on the phone" or "Puhleeeeze, can I just have one more cookie?"

A big reason kids can't explain why they feel compelled to perform rituals is that *it wasn't their idea to begin with.* It was and is OCD's idea. As we pointed out in Chapter 1, critical to understanding OCD is knowing that it's separate from your child. Your child doesn't *want* to perform this senseless act, and doing it is *no fun.* Here's what Andrew's morning looks like from this perspective—a view that is an important start toward understanding what OCD really looks like:

Andrew trotted down the stairs to the kitchen, carefully avoiding touching the banisters with his hands or brushing against them by staying right in the middle of the steps, because he knew OCD would make him feel really bad if he got near anything that could be dusty or dirty. The first thing he saw when he got to the table was that his mother had put out a spoon from the extra silverware, not the usual stuff. OCD made him stop in his tracks and rang a loud alarm that something was wrong. *Why was something different here?* OCD asked. *How could Andrew be sure it was clean if it hadn't just come out of the dishwasher?* OCD wanted to know. *Better be extra careful and not touch* anything—*it might not be safe, and if you make a wrong move, you'll be responsible for everyone getting sick, maybe dying,* said OCD. So Andrew cautiously pulled out his chair, holding his shirtsleeve over his hand to avoid direct contact, and sat down. As his mom brought out the milk and poured his juice, OCD pointed out that his napkin was on the right side of his bowl, not the left. *And what was that little speck on the edge of his bowl?* OCD added. *That juice glass didn't look as clean as it usually was when it came out of the dishwasher, did it?* OCD asked Andrew. *Had his mom accidentally given him a glass that his sister had already used and just rinsed out?* OCD made Andrew feel squirmy and more and more worried. *Maybe,* it said, *he better take a good look at the cereal. And what about the milk: was it fresh?* Andrew thought he should probably just look at the expiration date on the carton, but OCD warned him not to touch it till he was sure it was still fresh. Now he felt worse. If he got up, his mom would notice and give him that look. . . .

Knowing what your child is experiencing can help you determine what to do to help at any one time, as Part II of this book will show. To your child, OCD probably feels unstoppable right now. But OCD isn't a speeding train so much as a row of dominoes. It's a sequence of events, in which one leads to the next and then the next, with opportunities along the way to disrupt the sequence. When we break down that sequence into its components, you and your child will gain a better understanding of how you can keep OCD from toppling those dominoes. First, though, step back and take a more objective look at the big picture.

An Overview of Obsessions and Compulsions

The cardinal feature of OCD in young people is the need to neutralize obsessions by performing rituals. Unwanted thoughts and/or images (what we call obsessions) pop into the child's or teen's head, bringing with them unpleasant sensations ranging from worry to fear to disgust, shame, and guilt. Your son or daughter then performs some specific act (a compulsion or ritual) aimed at easing those sensations or reducing the chances that feared consequences will occur (that a loved one will get sick and die, for example). The rituals may be performed out in the open (such as washing) or secretly (such as counting mentally).

Almost everyone has behaviors that look a little like OCD but are so common as to be normal. Maybe you check your pocket for your keys several times before leaving home because you're afraid of locking yourself out. You probably don't do it to the point of making yourself an hour late for every appointment, though, and it doesn't seem strange or weird to you, and that's the distinction between normal behavior (too mild to diagnose, too common to be abnormal) and OCD.

> **WHAT TO SAY TO YOUR CHILD ABOUT OCD**
>
> "We know OCD isn't your idea and you'd make it go away if you could—that's why we're reading this book. Just remember how much trouble OCD causes you—it makes you late for school; it keeps you from playing at your friends' houses [substitute whatever impairment your child suffers]—and you'll be able to keep in mind that this is an illness. It's not your choice to have it, and we're going to make it better."

It can be difficult to distinguish between OCD and rituals that are a welcome part of daily life, such as bedtime songs, religious practices, and sports rituals. Normal worries, such as contamination fears, may also increase during times of stress, such as when someone in the family is sick or dying. Only when symptoms persist, make no sense, cause much distress, or interfere with functioning should they be considered OCD. You and your child may not have a hard time distinguishing between what's normal and what's OCD, because, as mentioned in Chapter 1, your child probably knows and can say that the obsessions and compulsions that plague him aren't normal. This isn't true of all kids, however, and that's why the criteria that doctors use to diagnose kids and teens don't require this insight to make a diagnosis. You can sharpen your own understanding of what is OCD and what is normal by reading about obsessions and compulsions here. Also, a child who is up to it can read Part I. You can pass the information along to a child who's not.

OCD takes a variety of forms. Your child may have obsessions that are exaggerated concerns shared by most children (such as fear of burglary resulting from leaving the front door unlocked). Or she may have highly unusual and illogical fears (such as loss of her soul due to failure to neutralize a sexual thought). Most kids and teens with OCD have both obsessions and compulsions, though very rarely a person with OCD may sometimes have only one or the other.

Your child's doctor will classify the type of OCD your child has based on compulsions rather than obsessions, because it's the compulsions that usually are easy to observe and cause the most trouble. Although many kids have more than one form of ritual, the predominant one typically determines how any individual's OCD symptoms are classified. So doctors describe their patients as washers, checkers, orderers, and so on. The table on the following page lists some common classifications of obsessions and compulsions; you'll find more details on each classification in the sections on obsessions and compulsions that follow.

WHAT TO SAY TO YOUR CHILD ABOUT OCD

"OCD comes in a lot of different flavors, just like ice cream. The kind you have may not be the same kind another kid has, but there are similarities that have helped scientists come up with ways that all kids can use to get rid of OCD."

Obsessions: Mental Hiccups

As mentioned before, obsessions are accompanied by an uncomfortable, distressing, or disturbing feeling that the child with OCD wants to get rid of—now. It's not unlike the thought, fear, or urge that we all have in response to something undesirable or dangerous. When we smell smoke, our inner alarm system goes off, telling us to beware of fire. But if we check out the house and then realize we're smelling the chimney smoke from the neighbor's fireplace, the alarm shuts off. Mostly, this kind of checking happens automatically, on the margins of awareness. Not so in OCD. Kids and teens (and adults) with OCD think they know from experience that obsessions won't go away without doing something to get rid of them.

When OCD causes your child to have an obsession, the thought, fear, or urge that comes with it doesn't go away when it would be obvious to most people that there's no danger and when your child has already taken the ordinary action in response. For example, if we can't avoid touching something really dirty, say, a public toilet in a gas station, most of us will feel the urge to wash our hands. But once we wash in a way that would be ordinary to most people, we stop feeling afraid that we're picking up germs. The fear of contamination and the urge to wash pass all by themselves, and we go on about our business without a second thought. We don't

Classifications of OCD

OCD Subtype	Obsessions	Common Compulsions	Example
Washing	Worries about dirt, germs, radiation, chemicals, environmental contaminants, etc.	Washing Cleaning	Shelly worries about HIV and won't use public restrooms. OCD makes her wash her hands according to specific rules.
Checking	Imagining having harmed self or others; being responsible for something bad happening	Checking	OCD has Billy worrying that he might have accidentally killed his sister, so he hides the knives and checks on her constantly.
Ordering/Arranging/ Symmetry	A need to have things even, balanced, or "just so"	Ordering/ arranging Touching Grooming	For no obvious reason, OCD requires Sam to have two pencils lined up exactly 6 inches apart before he can start his homework. Usually takes about 45 minutes, so he often skips homework.
Counting/Repeating	Magical numbers; a sense of "incompleteness"; urge to repeat	Counting Repeating Grooming Touching	OCD has Eva do everything six times or in multiples of six: rereading, hair brushing, washing her hands, speaking words. Totally disabling.
Scrupulosity	Intrusive sexual thoughts or urges; excessive religious or moral doubt; a need to tell, ask, confess	Praying Reassurance seeking	Even though he's happily heterosexual, OCD has Adam worrying that because he looks at a boy, he might be gay. Mostly he looks down or up, but when he can't he says prayers until OCD lets go.
Hoarding	Fear of losing something	Can't throw things away Checks to see if he or she has thrown something away	OCD tells Lorraine that if she can't find what she needs, something terrible will happen, and because what that something is is unknown, she can't throw anything out.

have to obsess; we resolve fear of contamination automatically through reasonable thinking and ordinary behavior. In contrast, the fear of contamination in OCD is exaggerated and refuses to pass out of mind, even with excessive washing.

WHAT TO SAY TO YOUR CHILD ABOUT OCD

"It must be so hard to do what you feel like you have to do and then find out that OCD still won't go away. I know you're doing your best to stop feeling afraid, or anxious, or just plain old bad. If you're like most kids with OCD, you'd like nothing better than to learn how to make those thoughts and bad feelings go away."

Why this happens is less important right now than getting an inside look at obsessions so you can understand your child's experience. (What is happening in the brain during obsessions and compulsions is discussed in Chapter 3.) Here are some insights that will help.

1. *Obsessions are not just a little too much worry about real threats.* Janie thinks that if she touches anything greasy, she'll transfer it to her mother, who will then be unable to get rid of it, and the grease will "turn into" a disease that will kill her mother. Sure, it's possible for people to transfer germs to each other, but the chances that this occurrence will lead to a terminal illness are slim to none. And yes, lack of cleanliness can mean that germs hang around longer than you want them to, but "grease" by itself doesn't cause disease. Still, the reasonable concern (that being exposed to germs can make you sick, to name a typical one) at the core of many obsessions sometimes can make drawing the line between normal worry and obsession tricky. On the other hand, even fastidious people can easily tell the difference between ordinary cleanliness and OCD.

Kids and parents can also be confused by the fact that we consider some obsessional behavior perfectly normal. Experts tell us that it's not only normal but necessary for little kids to indulge in repetitive behaviors to master specific aspects of normal development. You might remember you or your child insisting on an elaborate bedtime ritual to ease the fear of being isolated from parents and in the dark at night. Or maybe you know a child who liked to arrange and rearrange his collection of baseball cards. The difference between these healthy attempts to mature and adapt to the world and OCD, however, is that the normal obsessiveness disappears or changes into something else during the process of growing up, whereas OCD seems strangely out of sync with normal development.

Although children with OCD may not differ significantly in number or type of superstitions, they have a lot more marked early ritualistic behaviors than normal kids, even when behaviors that resemble primary OCD symptoms are discounted. Parents might roll their eyes in impatience at a preschooler's requests for a certain ritual, but they wouldn't view the behavior as troubling, whereas when OCD appears, it's pretty clear that the obsessions and accompanying rituals don't seem normal. For example, kids with OCD might want not just a bedtime story but a strict sequence of bedtime events. Some will eat only a very few foods prepared in limited ways, taking the term "picky eater" to new lengths. You may recall that it was only over time that you started to realize that these were not just little personality quirks in your child but a growing pattern of obsessive–compulsive behavior.

Kids with OCD can prove to themselves that their worries are not realistic by gradually facing what they fear and seeing how harmless it actually is. But they need skills such as those in Part II to help them do it. They can't be expected to "get real" and "be sensible" and "stop all this nonsense" on command.

2. *Obsessions tend to expand, morph, and multiply when left untreated.* The obsessions that plague kids with OCD are not about simple common fears such as fear of the dark or of strangers. They usually have something to do with contamination, illness, or death, other dangers, keeping things "just so," and sometimes, especially as kids get older, sex or religion. There's also a whole category of obsessions about numbers and another about hoarding. There are all kinds of variations on these themes, as described later. You should be aware, however, that two-thirds of kids with OCD have more than one type of obsession and that new obsessions frequently arise, disappear, and change their appearance. When OCD goes untreated, many kids end up having or having had all the typical types of obsessions and compulsions by the time they are adults. That's a good reason to start working on the program in Part II as soon as you can.

3. *What OCD is saying to the child may not be obvious.* Janie's obsession—that any grease she touches will infect and eventually kill her mother—started when they visited a fast food restaurant and her mother joked that the food was so greasy it would probably make the people who ate there turn into grease balls. OCD popped up and told Janie that maybe she'd better not eat (she picked at her food) and that perhaps grease was bad not only for her but for others in her family, too. Most kids would laugh this off, and the thought would recede automatically, but with Janie, that stop signal is on the fritz, and the thoughts (obsessions) came on in a rush and persisted. Now Janie won't eat anything OCD says contains oil, insists that the stovetop at home be wiped clean 10 times after dinner, washes her own hands repeatedly after every meal, washes her hands even if she just touches something in the kitchen or anywhere that food is prepared, and has even started avoiding grocery stores. Without asking, Jamie's mother would have no idea that avoidance of the supermarket was related to the same urge that makes Janie obsessed with cleanliness in the kitchen.

4. *Sometimes obsessions develop after a major stressful experience, but that doesn't mean the obsession is caused by the experience or is a natural reaction to it.* In some cases kids begin to develop certain obsessions connected with a particularly stressful experience in their lives. Kids who experience the death of a loved one may develop obsessions about death (or the cause of death of their loved one), those who witness a crime may start to obsess about being victimized or causing that kind of crime, and so forth. On the other hand, most kids experience stressful events, and just because OCD starts up doesn't mean that it has anything to do with a child's life experiences. More often than not, OCD starts insidiously without any rhyme or reason.

5. *Obsessions are so intrusive that they interfere with many parts of life.* Donny was sitting in his fourth-grade classroom when he glanced up at the clock and saw that only an hour remained in the school day, which triggered the obsession that he'd miss the school bus and be stranded, alone, outside the school because he didn't know what time it was. Of course, he did know what time it was, and this had never happened and never would happen, as he was by temperament a cautious, attentive youngster. Nonetheless, OCD said that he might be wrong about the time, so he'd better keep close track of the time so he could get out of the building and not miss the bus. So he'd check the clock over and over again, even though he knew what time it was—by the way, we call this kind of obsession "doubting," and it can show up in all kinds of situations. Before he knew it, Donny was trapped in a spiral of thoughts about how he would be able to pack up his backpack and fight through the crowds in the hall and get to the bus on time. At first, OCD got going only at the end of the day, but later the obsession began running in the morning, and checking started earlier and earlier in the day. Donny's mother was perplexed when she got a call from his teacher saying her formerly alert, conscientious student was so spaced out during the day that his grades were beginning to suffer. Donny's situation is pretty typical of the kind of nonsense OCD pulls: a doubting obsession about time and a clock-checking ritual. Unless you knew to look for OCD, this one would be easy to mistake for separation anxiety, which is why it is important to get educated about OCD and to have a doctor who has done the same.

Obsessional thoughts can take center stage in a kid's mind, shoving what's going on in the classroom into the wings. They can interfere with homework or test taking or chores or even fun activities, like watching a movie or playing a board game. To parents and teachers, a child stuck in obsessional thoughts (or mental compulsions; see later in the chapter) may seem like he's developed an attention problem. Kids with OCD have been accused of being lazy, of spending all their time "daydreaming," or of being unmotivated. They may start to do poorly in school or lose friends due to their apparent distraction all the time. Because other people don't know what's going on in their heads, they may be suspected of having ADHD instead of OCD (see page 46). Mean-

> **WHAT TO SAY TO YOUR CHILD ABOUT OCD**
>
> "Do those worries that are bugging you at home bother you in other places too? Are they making it hard for you to pay attention to your teacher or get your work done in class? Do they come up when you're playing with your friends or when you're at someone else's house? I'm really proud of you for trying to deal with OCD on your own, but if you help me understand where and how OCD bothers you, I might be able to help."

while, the child with OCD is struggling mightily to fight off what many kids call "dumb," "goofy," "ridiculous," or "insane" obsessions while worrying that his inability to do so means he's "crazy." Doesn't leave much time for the business of growing up, does it?

Typical Obsessions in Children

Fear of Contamination

The most common obsessions, contamination obsessions, tell the child that she, or someone she loves, will get contaminated by germs and that this in turn will lead to getting sick or even dying. But children we've known have also been obsessed about contamination with dirt, ink, paint, excrement, chemicals, radiation, pollution or other environmental toxins, and all kinds of other substances. Current events and other news provide fertile ground for contamination fears. For example, in the last couple of decades the fear of AIDS has shown up in OCD, with obsessions about contamination from blood or other bodily fluids.

At some point in the course of their illness, about 80% of kids become obsessed with one or another contamination fear. Most of the time what they do to minimize OCD is to spend lots of time trying to avoid contamination and, when it can't be avoided, lots of time washing or cleaning, as discussed in the section on compulsions. Because kids are usually ashamed of their obsessions and compulsions and go to great lengths to keep them a secret, you may have no idea that the compulsions are even being triggered by OCD. Signs of contamination obsessions to watch for include hands that have gotten dry, red, chapped, or cracked from washing; in school, kids who ask to go to the restroom all the time may be going there to wash their hands over and over. Or kids may refuse to go to certain places (that OCD says are dirty) or won't use certain restrooms for reasons that make no sense. Leaving books at the front steps or washing textbooks is a cardinal sign of contamination obsessions. Some kids who fear contamination may look dirty or sloppy, rather than overly fastidious, because they're afraid to contaminate certain body parts and therefore won't touch them at all.

Fear of Harm, Illness, or Death

Obsessions about harm can take forms other than contamination. OCD may get kids to worry about their own safety or that of their parents or other loved ones. They may find themselves constantly agonizing over the possibility that they or a family member will be poisoned, be killed by a falling object, have a car accident, or be the victim of a natural disaster, such as a tornado, that the youngster with OCD should have prevented or warned about. Even though it makes no sense to anyone, this common obsession is the fear that they have harmed or will harm someone else. It is common to find an adult with OCD driving around and around the block because OCD tells her that she might have hit a pedestrian. We've seen this with a child whose obsession was that he might have run over a cat on his bike—he knew it hadn't happened but couldn't stop the obsession and spent hours looking for the injured cat. OCD told another youngster that his dad would die in a car accident if the child didn't tell him at least seven times each morning to wear his seat belt. Because we all worry about those we love, these obsessions are particularly hard to address, unless you remember that they are OCD, not reality.

Obsessions with Numbers

OCD sometimes says that only certain numbers are safe—or that certain numbers are bad, or that things need to be done a certain number of times for no good reason except that that's what OCD says. Young boys in particular seem to fall prey to these obsessions, for which counting is the ritual. Number obsessions interfere with every aspect of life, because there's almost nothing that can't be done more than once. Imagine how hard life must be for a child who thinks he has to do everything 4 times or in multiples of 4. Picture trying to play a musical instrument, participate in sports, or learn to dance if every number you use has to be divisible by 4 or you have to do everything 4 times. Imagine the burden of having to chew everything 4, 8, or 12 times, wash your hands 4 times, close a door 4 times. Your child with OCD may know what it feels like to have to beg you to read not 1 more page of a bedtime story but 4 more pages or to reread the same page 4 times. If you see repeating rituals or avoidance behaviors that seem to involve "good" or "bad" numbers, you can bet that counting is one of the things that OCD is up to with your child.

Obsessions with Sex

Not surprisingly, sexual obsessions are particularly difficult for kids to talk about. What is really clear is that, without exception, kids find them very disturbing. Kids with such obsessions can end up weighed down with guilt and shame—so much so that some will go to huge lengths to neutralize these thoughts. Sexual obsessions are often connected to feeling sinful and get all tangled up in religion. They not uncommonly involve homosexual content, even though the youngster is entirely heterosexual. Sometimes, sexual obsessions can involve family members: all deeply disturbing stuff. It is especially important to point out that sexual obsessions, like all other obsessions, are just mental hiccups and have no personal meaning, value, or reality. They definitely don't warrant child abuse evaluations or intensive psychotherapy to resolve deep conflicts about sex. They are just OCD, nothing more.

"Just So," Hoarding, and Other Obsessions

As you can see on the checklist on pages 266–267 at the back of the book, there are a variety of other obsessions. Many involve urges or images or just uncomfortable feelings rather than discrete thoughts. For example, although hoarding often involves fear of harm associated with not having something that OCD says is essential to survival, it just as often involves the fear of losing something, without any feared consequences. Sometimes this is felt as major unease or discomfort, not as fear. There is no feared consequence to be neutralized, just an urge that nags and must be satisfied. Other children experience "just so" urges that provoke balancing, evening, touching, or tapping rituals. Repeating and counting rituals often involve "just so" urges. For example, OCD had Leah brush her hair in multiples of six, striving for perfect balance on each side—which took 30 minutes on a good day, hours on a bad day. When asked "Why?" she responded "I just have to." And, in this instance, that's exactly true. OCD is just a (for now) seemingly irresistible urge.

Because these forms of OCD mostly involve compulsions as much as or more than discrete obsessions, we discuss them in the next section, but you should know that it is impossible to detail all the forms that OCD may take. That's why we will make a very careful map of OCD that is specific to your child and use this map as a guide to breaking the rules OCD has set for your child and family.

Compulsions: Trying to Make It All Better

The essential fact about compulsions is part of the definition of the word. Kids with OCD feel they *have to* perform certain actions to ease the disturbing thoughts, feelings, or urges that define obsessions. OCD tells them these actions must be done according to certain rules or in a very particular way. When the child does perform a ritual the way OCD demands, he feels better—at least temporarily. As we'll see in detail in Chapter 3, playing OCD's game this way only makes the obsessions occur more and more often, demanding more and more rituals, until obsessions and compulsions take up a big chunk of a child's daily life.

Sometimes the compulsions are obviously intended to prevent the feared event from happening. Washing hands repeatedly is the classic example of a compulsive ritual performed in response to a fear of contamination. Janie's avoidance of the grocery store might not seem connected to an obsession about contamination unless you knew that OCD had her deathly afraid that she might encounter some kind of cooking oil, have an allergic reaction, and die on the spot. Avoiding people, places, or things connected with the obsession is a very common element in most compulsions. Janie avoids all oils, the grocery store, and even people involved with storing, selling, and cooking food.

As is shown in the table in this chapter, compulsions, like obsessions, tend to cluster together. Ritualized washing is the most common compulsion in children and adolescents and is typically performed to decrease discomfort associated with contamination obsessions. For example, individuals who fear contact with "AIDS germs" clean themselves and their environment excessively to prevent contracting AIDS themselves or spreading it to others. Most children with washing rituals can identify a specific disaster that will occur if they refrain from compulsive washing. For some kids with washing rituals, a sense of being contaminated all by itself generates tremendous discomfort. A good example is feeling "sticky." To decrease this distress, OCD compels them to engage in washing rituals. This a good example of why it is important to investigate OCD carefully, as there is no feared consequence that provokes washing—you know only if you ask.

Another common compulsion is repetitive checking, which is typically performed to prevent a future catastrophe. Children and adolescents with lock-checking rituals may worry more about losing items out of their lockers at school, whereas an adult would worry about the car being stolen, but the basic phenomenon is the same. Youngsters with obsessions that they might have harmed someone or somehow will be responsible for something bad happening will repeatedly check to make sure that the feared consequence has not happened, without realizing that doing rituals will increase rather than decrease anxiety in the long run—a crucial fact discussed a little further on.

Children who have repeating rituals are similar to checkers in that they, too, are typically driven by the wish to prevent bad things from happening; however, they often differ from checkers in that their rituals are unrelated logically to their feared consequences. For example, it is logical (if excessive) to check the front door lock many times if you fear a burglary but illogical to walk up and down the stairs repeatedly to prevent a loved one's death in a motor vehicle accident. Other children with repeating rituals have no feared consequence. Rather, the repeating rituals may be more "tic-like"—there is no feared consequence to be avoided but simply an uncomfortable feeling or urge to be alleviated. For example, it is not uncommon to see prolonged grooming, stepping, touching, or other nonsensical repetitive behavior that is done for no other reason than that OCD insists on it.

Ordering, arranging, and counting can follow from obsessions that involve feared consequences, from an uncomfortable feeling that things must be "just so," or from the urge to have things symmetrical, evened up, or balanced. Some kids feel they have to get dressed in a very precise order. Or they have to eat their breakfast in a specific sequence or eat just the right amount of cereal. Once at school, they may have to check and recheck their answers on a test or write and erase their names on their classwork over and over. Sometimes they just to have repeat certain common movements—walking, getting in and out of chairs, sharpening pencils, reading a page, even asking questions in class—in a certain way and for a prescribed number of times or it "doesn't feel right," and they have to start over and can't move on to the next goal. Likewise, a child might feel he has to have everything on his body symmetrical. He might tie his shoelaces over and over until they look exactly balanced and even. She might feel that objects in her bedroom or classroom have to be arranged so they seem symmetrical and balanced. The way the child moves may have to be even: taking steps of the same length, speaking with the same stress on each syllable.

Checking and repeating may be a manifestation of a more general pattern of *obsessive doubting* that compels the child to make sure that he or she didn't hurt someone's feelings, cheat on a test, desire something morally repugnant, or commit a sin. Such children may anxiously plague their parents with compulsive confessions of imagined misdeeds or bad thoughts and requests for reassurance regarding what OCD has them believing is of paramount moral or religious concern. In some children OCD takes on a specifically religious form, with repetitive praying or worries about imagined sins (religious scrupulosity); in other children, the concern is more with breaking moral commandments, such as somehow cheating on a test or telling a lie (moral scrupulosity). Either way, when coupled with doubting, scrupulosity is often challenging, in part because it overlaps with normal beliefs held by the child, the parents, and possibly a therapist. We'll have more to say about this later.

Finally, hoarding is a rare but important subtype of OCD in kids, as it is in adults. Most kids with hoarding don't collect things. Rather, they avoid discarding items they encounter in everyday life (e.g., newspapers, string) for fear of not having them available in the future. Over long periods of time, consistent avoidance of discarding can result in overwhelming accumulations of junk, even in the absence of active collecting rituals. Hoarded material can also vary from items of some monetary value (such as complete sets of the latest game cards) to those that are worthless (chicken bones or empty milk containers). It can be hard to make that critical distinction between normal behavior and OCD when the hoarded material can be viewed as "collectibles." A child who obsessively loves and so collects action figures would routinely discuss his collections with his friends at school who had similar collections in their own homes. However, another child with OCD being treated for hoarding felt that he had to keep the ripped cardboard boxes that the action figures came in, as well as the wrapping paper that covered the boxes if they were given as presents, and he had four of each figure "in case something happened to the main ones." The collector had fun and thought it all normal; the child with hoarding hated it but couldn't stop.

Doctors and scientists used to believe that some kids with OCD had obsessions without compulsions, but we now think that in almost all of those cases what's really going on is that the compulsions are mental. Some kids do all their checking or counting in their heads. No one sees them do it, although a parent or teacher certainly might notice that the child seems distracted and unable to attend to schoolwork or other tasks at hand. As with obsessions, compulsions can evolve or be replaced by other compulsions over time.

Whatever they are, compulsions can take up lots of time, making it hard for kids to attend to the business of both work and play. Kids with OCD can end up missing lots of school because their morning rituals take longer and longer every day or have to be started over when not completed just right.

Triggers: Little Things That Have a Big Impact

For both parents and their kids, it's pretty hard to fathom how an obsession pops up, leading to that cascade of toppled dominoes that define an attack of OCD. What triggers obsession in kids with OCD? Chapter 3 sheds some light on how OCD episodes unfold by showing what goes on in the brain. For now, though, it's important to understand the kinds of things that can serve as OCD's cue to seize the moment.

It's almost as if OCD puts the world under a magnifying glass. When the obsessions a child experiences have to do with contamination, for example, a speck of dirt spied out of the corner of his eye can zoom in to fill his vision, as if a telephoto lens had suddenly been trained on it. OCD controls that lens. There's often no room for anything else—just OCD. The child is neither choosing to focus on the speck nor failing to fight the fear that arises when he sees it. Kids with OCD do fight it. They just don't have the necessary skills to win the battle, so they resort to rituals to make the obsession go away. Until they learn the skills we teach in this program, there's no other way out, and this, of course, keeps the child trapped.

The fact is, a wide variety of stimuli can set off OCD. Andrew's mom had followed the "rules" set by her son's OCD: She had washed everything in sight so Andrew wouldn't start obsessing about whether eating breakfast would cause him to pick up a germ that would make him—and his mom—sick. It never occurred to her that anything new at the table would trigger Andrew's OCD. But, as you could see from knowing what went on in Andrew's mind, a simple thing like a different spoon led to a series of thoughts that made Andrew fear contamination.

As you'll continue to learn throughout this book, it's only by not playing OCD's game that a child can neutralize the triggers of OCD. It's all about expectations. Trying to help her son, Andrew's mom made sure everything was clean and made sure Andrew *knew* everything was clean by keeping the breakfast routine consistent. Unfortunately, that only meant that when OCD's expectations were not met—even in a tiny way like using a different spoon—the fear of contamination would naturally be triggered. If everything was the way it was "supposed to be," he would stay germ free. The minute the tableau was disrupted, that guarantee was threatened.

So what kinds of things can trigger OCD? Before a child learns the techniques in this book, a trigger can be anything outside the routine, even if it seems as though it's not related directly to the object of the child's obsessions. Andrew can fear contamination at breakfast not just when he sees any evidence of uncleanliness but when he sees *any* change. OCD makes Billy feel he has to get his socks even and "just right" before he can go to school. He'd like to quit wearing socks, but it is too cold (he lives in Maine), so he asks his Mom if his socks are OK over and over. The obsessions that bother Amy involve the need to start the day with a sequence of prayers in multiples of three—or she'll have a bad day. She can't avoid getting up, so she gets up hours before she has to. OCD makes Grant worry that he might have lost something he needs, and he knows that 2 or 3 hours will be spent looking, even though he doesn't know what he's looking for. Getting rid of trash cans doesn't help; he tried, but OCD made him look under the bed and even in the garbage disposal. Sam hates intrusive sexual thoughts that arise when he sees other boys—he really likes girls and isn't gay—but trying to make the thoughts go away by avoiding looking at his male friends makes them worse, and his friends now think he's gone nuts. And the more detailed and

WHAT TO SAY TO YOUR CHILD ABOUT OCD

"I bet it feels really bad when OCD arises. Every time you have to use the bathroom, OCD jumps in and takes over. What a pain. How would it be if we came up with some ways for you to shrug OCD off before it gets going instead of getting lost in it?"

complicated the routine becomes, the more difficult it is to avoid the situations that trigger obsessions and compulsions.

Thinking of OCD as being triggered by something—like someone pushing over the first domino in a row—is a helpful way to understand the way OCD works, because from the outside it can look as though a boy or girl was going along just fine when suddenly something changed and the child started performing a nonsensical ritual out of the blue. It's important to be aware that OCD has a certain logic, even though it may not look that way. For example, there are many possible triggers for OCD that are not visible to an outside observer. In one, the child's obsessions and compulsions aren't set off by a reminder or stimulus, because the child isn't obsessed with a fear of being contaminated or of losing things or of causing an accident or injury. Some kids with OCD just feel compelled to do things a certain number of times, in a certain order, or in a balanced, symmetrical way. Similarly, some kids blink, tap objects, or make some other motion that has no real purpose over and over, for no particular reason except that OCD makes them do it. Obsessions and compulsions aren't triggered in these kids by some reminder. Rather, they feel that they have to perform their rituals until things "feel right." These repetitive, orderly actions can pop up anywhere, anytime, and over time they're likely to spread to more and more areas of the child's life and take up more and more time. Parents in this case need to be aware simply that the child feels no control over these actions and really means it when she says "I just have to." She has no other explanation for why the behavior is necessary; she only knows she gets (temporary) relief from OCD by doing the ritual.

For parents and kids, trying to understand why a child feels driven to perform a ritual—what triggers that action—can be extremely helpful, *but only to a point.* Knowing that a different spoon on the table can set off a cascade of fearful thoughts about contamination will help Andrew's mother empathize with her son and respond constructively, instead of just getting aggravated. Bringing his fears of contamination out in the light of day so he can label them as OCD, not his thoughts, will help Andrew know that he's not "crazy," but that OCD sure is silly. Andrew and his mom can end up pulling together to fight OCD as a result of this understanding.

But when it's impossible to know what triggers OCD—when OCD just pops up—it is essential to drop the search to identify a trigger. We've discovered that *changing the behavior* is the key to stopping the sequence of events that is OCD. Then the thoughts (obsessions) will diminish, and so will the potency of the triggers.

Not only is it a waste of energy to try to figure out what triggers obsessions in your child, but you should also know without a doubt that *it's not you.* Earlier we said that Janie's obsession with contamination from oil started when her mother made a joke about how greasy the food was in the restaurant they were in. *This does not mean that Janie's mother's comment* caused *Janie to have OCD—or that Janie's mother can prevent obsessions by being careful about what she says.* OCD is irrational and inconsistent. We scientists don't know why certain obsessions occur in certain kids or why OCD might rear its obnoxious head in some situations and not others. (Some kids, for example, don't experience obsessions at school, whereas others experience the same types of obsessions only at school—and we have no way of determining why.) The problem is a broken switch in the brain that keeps OCD running on and on like a car on a racetrack with no exit. So don't expend your valuable energy trying to guard what you say. In Part II we'll give you some terrific ideas for how to verbally support your child's successes in talking back to OCD and how to talk to your child about the other, good things in his life so that OCD gets yanked out of center stage.

Consequences: OCD Expands Its Territory, and Life Narrows

What most kids and parents don't realize is that "obeying" OCD makes it greedy for more. Again, Chapter 3 explains further, but the point here is that the short-term relief that kids feel they get from obsessions when they perform OCD's rituals doesn't last. OCD not only comes back but also comes back for more and more over time. A girl who once felt it was sufficient to wash her hands 5 times after lunch now ends up late for her first afternoon class because OCD makes her feel she needs to do it 10 and then 15 times. A child who used to hoard soda cans now heeds OCD's command to hoard bottles, too. OCD tells a girl who used to rearrange her dolls in a neat row every morning that she now has to do the same thing with all her books before she goes to school.

Before they know it, many kids with OCD find that they're hardly doing anything *they* want to do; they're spending all their time doing what OCD wants them to do. Life isn't much fun anymore. Some kids drop out of organized sports and Scouts and other group activities because they don't fit in when OCD is tagging along. Some lose friends and end up pretty isolated because other kids don't want to wait around while they perform all their rituals. Or the other kids just find they're competing with OCD for the child's attention, and that's not much of a friendship.

If OCD intrudes into the school day, the child may have a pretty hard time sticking to the schedule imposed by the teacher. She may have difficulty completing any assignment or test within the time allotted. OCD's demands for order may disrupt the classroom and impinge on classmates' rights. The child may be so distracted mentally that she stops hearing the teacher or participating in class—or she may insist on asking the same questions over and over. As the box on page 44 shows, kids with OCD tend to have the intelligence it takes to succeed in school—but OCD gets in the way.

WHAT TO SAY TO YOUR CHILD ABOUT OCD

"I'm worried that you don't have as much fun as you used to. What do you feel like you don't have time for anymore? Why don't we make a list of all the things you love to do that you'd like to start doing again? Then we'll start figuring out how to take the time back from OCD and return it to you. Once we get rid of OCD, it'll be fun to figure out how to use all that free time."

On top of losing time and being distracted from the rest of life, kids with OCD can end up going to great lengths to avoid OCD triggers, an avoidance that can cause additional problems. If OCD makes a child feel bad about her inability to finish a test, she may start to make excuses for staying home from school, threatening her academic performance even further. A child who is embarrassed by the compulsion to click his tongue when he speaks to people may become more and more mute, isolating himself more than ever. The long rituals a teenager feels compelled to perform before leaving the house may turn her into a recluse. It's as if OCD not only occupies a greater and greater part of the child's mind and energy but also begins to claim more and more of the child's life. Most kids with OCD are demoralized by it—many become depressed, which means two problems, not just one. The cure: Get rid of OCD.

Diagnosing OCD

Before using the program in this book, even if it's pretty plain that your child is experiencing obsessions and compulsions like the ones just described, it's wise to see a knowledgeable professional, whether that means starting with your pediatrician or school psychologist or finding a therapist or child and adolescent psychiatrist. You may already have followed this path, and your child may already be working with a therapist. If not, and if you don't have a firm diagnosis of OCD and whatever other problems may be present, now is a good time to seek one out.

Like any mental, emotional, or behavioral illness, OCD requires skill and attention to diagnose accurately. It's always best to determine, when seeking an evaluation, that the person consulted has experience not just with OCD but with OCD in children and teenagers. Most kids with OCD have had it for a long time before they receive a correct diagnosis, in part because mental health professionals are not up to speed in the care of young people with OCD. OCD can also be confused with other illnesses, such as ADHD, as mentioned earlier and discussed further later. And even with a correct diagnosis, the wait for good treatment such as the program we walk you through in Part II can be long, which is one of the reasons we wrote this book. The resources section at the back gives some tips for finding mental health professionals who are experienced with the type of program you'll learn in Part II. Follow these guidelines if you have not yet consulted a professional or if you're not sure your child has received an appropriate diagnosis so far.

A lot of kids get worried—as if they don't already have enough worries!—about seeing a doctor for their problem. Does this mean they're crazy after all? Of course not. It means that they and their parents have decided it's time to find out exactly what's wrong and what can be done about it. It is just like going to the doctor for a chronic stomachache. It should mean the beginning of an end to your worries, not a whole bunch of new ones.

So what should you expect? Of course, the exact approach will vary depending on whom you consult. But if you see a psychologist or psychiatrist for a full evaluation, the doctor will probably want to meet with both your child and you and sometimes the rest of the immediate family. If the first interview involves all of you, you'll probably feel relieved to hear the doctor explaining that OCD is an illness and that the way the child has been thinking, feeling, and acting not only isn't his fault but doesn't make him crazy. If the doctor meets with your son or daughter alone, the main topic of conversation should be what's bothering the child: how OCD is interfering in the child's life, how much time it takes up, how the child views it, and how upset the child is by it.

If you go to a doctor who ends up focusing on how you all get along with each other or who just wants to play games and get to know your child and who doesn't listen to you about concentrating on cognitive-behavioral treatment of OCD, then you might be in the wrong place. It's not that the doctor isn't good; it is just that OCD requires specialized care. A doctor who at least has heard of this program—or, even better, who uses it already—is the best choice to make a diagnosis of OCD.

Many doctors use rating scales and checklists to figure out exactly what's going on, how severe the problem is, and how long it's been around. This will help them determine whether the child might have OCD and what kind of treatment might help, if so. One of these checklists is included at the back of the book to help you take an inventory of all the obsessions and compulsions that OCD is foisting on the child. One of the scales that professionals use has been adapted for use as a tool to measure progress in the program in Part II.

A doctor should make a diagnosis of OCD if and only if the criteria from the American Psychiatric Association's *Diagnostic and Statistical Manual of Mental Disorders* are met. Although it is not strictly necessary for the child to distinguish OCD from normal thinking and behavior (although most do), the *DSM* says the following about OCD:

- The child has to have either obsessions or compulsions that fit the descriptions given in this chapter.
- The child knows the obsessions are coming from his own mind.
- The child tries to ignore or eliminate them by performing some ritual but knows that the rituals aren't normal.
- The obsessions and compulsions aren't caused by another diagnosable condition.
- Perhaps most important of all, the obsessions and compulsions are causing distress and interfering with the child's life.

The doctor will take into account everything learned from interviews with the child and family; from teachers, if the OCD is causing problems at school; and from any checklists or questionnaires. He or she will keep in mind certain things we know about kids with OCD that are listed in the box on page 44, and he or she will also be aware of the following factors that can make an accurate diagnosis difficult.

Your child doesn't have to fit the following description to have OCD, but here are a few things that are typical of kids with OCD:

- For boys, the obsessions and compulsions started at a pretty young age, say second or third grade. Boys are also likely to have ordering and arranging rituals driven by the need to have things even, balanced, or "just so" as their main type of obsession and compulsion.
- Girls' obsessions and compulsions are more likely to have started during high school, and they're more likely to have the fear and worry types of obsessions.
- Although more common in younger boys, both boys and girls are more likely to have problems such as ADHD or a tic disorder than children without OCD.
- Girls more than boys might also have problems with anxiety and depression.
- Both boys and girls with OCD are likely to be of average or above-average intelligence.
- Although the onset of OCD may seem to be, and in fact may be, connected to a specific, often traumatic, incident such as the death of a loved one, parents' divorce, or a move to a new location, it is not clear that stressful events are any more common in children with OCD than in those without OCD, and, in any case, looking back to figure out what historically caused OCD isn't helpful in getting better.

The Challenges of Diagnosing OCD

- *There are exceptions to every rule.* OCD can begin at any age, though it most commonly starts before the teen years and, with OCD that starts in adulthood, in the 20s. Rarely does OCD start after age 35 or before age 5, though OCD has been reported as early as age 2. I once met a 2½-year-old girl who had to rearrange her toys in a very specific way, and her mother, who had OCD, said she had been doing it since she was only 9 months old. Is this OCD? Is it the same illness as in someone whose OCD began as a teenager? Perhaps; perhaps not. One problem with identifying OCD in very young children is that they can't tell us about it. We just don't know exactly what OCD might look like in someone who is too young to talk and too young to think the way older kids think. In toddlers and preschoolers, doctors sometimes can't help confusing OCD with other problems, such as autism, that also involve repeating certain actions. With very young children, we typically end up treating the symptoms as best we can with CBT and, less often, medications, and just waiting until the diagnostic picture clarifies as the child grows up.

- *There may be more than one type of OCD.* Although boys seem to develop OCD at an earlier age than girls, by the time they're teenagers the number of boys and girls with OCD is about equal. What this and the other differences listed in the box mean is that OCD probably has a few different "types" (just as there are different forms and causes of arthritis) and that these types (and their causes) may have something to do with the age at which OCD starts. The good news is that researchers are hot on the trail of these different types, and, once these are understood, improvements in treatment will likely occur.

• *We can't find much link between ethnic background or geographical location and OCD.* The chance of having OCD appears to be remarkably similar all over the world, which is one of the characteristics of a brain disorder. So as far as we can tell, an Italian German American child who lives in North Carolina is just as likely to have OCD as his Asian American bunkmate in summer camp who hails from Oregon. On the other hand, whether a child comes for treatment seems to have something to do with cultural factors relating to identifying OCD as a problem and with willingness to come for treatment and to participate in research. For example, African American children, who appear to have the same chance of having OCD as European American children, are rarely seen in OCD clinics for reasons that we need to understand if we are going to do a better job of extending the benefits of the latest effective treatments to all children.

• *Each kid with OCD is unique.* Temperament (usual mood), personality (temperament plus life story), age, family and culture (background), knowledge about OCD, and thinking abilities all affect how a child thinks about and can talk about OCD. This means each youngster with OCD is unique, and that means we doctors have to look and listen very hard to find out exactly how OCD is messing up a child's life. The more kids tell us, the more we can help all kids with OCD. So we need to keep working together. Given the stigma that accompanies any mental disorder, I often like to point out that each of us is the product of billions of years of evolution— there is no one like you, and it took a very long time to make you. No matter our temperament or personal story, each of us deserves deep respect and the kindness that comes with it, and that's where this program begins.

• *Some of OCD's symptoms can look a lot like the symptoms of other mental disorders.* OCD can be easy to confuse with other disorders, especially other anxiety disorders. Some anxiety disorders also have nonsensical fears at their center. Although they are different from OCD, they sometimes look on the surface like OCD. For example, people who have a specific phobia—think fear of snakes or heights, for example—are usually afraid of one or two things or situations, and they ease their fears by avoiding those things, not by performing rituals. Despite these distinctions, there's a chance that a doctor could mistake one disorder for the other—or even for another anxiety disorder—unless he or she is experienced in working with kids with OCD.

Let's say your child has a fear of getting a bad grade on a test and spends a lot of time worrying about grades and, maybe, checking answers on tests. That fear may be a specific phobia called *test anxiety.* Or it could be a sign of social anxiety—the worry that she'll embarrass herself in front of classmates. Or it might turn out to be just one of all kinds of worries she feels and may go along with a desire to do everything perfectly. A child with generalized anxiety disorder might worry incessantly about getting into college and having a good job and so spend extra hours studying for tests, but this is an example of an exaggerated normal fear associated with perfectionism, not OCD. Or it could be OCD characterized by doubting as the obsession and by repeating and checking rituals.

How would a doctor know? If your child was pretending to be sick whenever a test was scheduled so she wouldn't have to go to school, many doctors might say the fact that she's avoiding tests means she has test anxiety, a kind of social phobia. If they probed further, they might discover that she was staying home from school because she's scared of having to talk in front of the class, another feature of social anxiety. But if you're reading this book, your child probably doesn't care more than normal about tests and can talk in class without any problem. Instead, her OCD is telling her not to use the bathroom because it is contaminated, and because that's pretty hard to do over a long school day, she finds ways to stay home. Or maybe it is saying something bad will happen if she uses the number 4, and of course 4 is in her locker combination and all her math tests. Missing school and other ways of avoiding things that trigger OCD is often one of the big things that causes problems in her life. As we said, OCD can be a very slippery character. The only way to know whether what bugs your child is OCD is for the doctor to ask and for your child to tell the doctor exactly how OCD makes her life harder.

As mentioned earlier, OCD is occasionally misdiagnosed as ADHD, especially in a child whose compulsions are all mental. When your mind is tied up with relentless obsessions or getting through the counting or listing rituals that OCD demands—or when you're just trying to think of something else to avoid getting trapped by obsessions—you don't have much brainpower left to pay attention to your math or science. Still, ADHD is pretty easy to distinguish from OCD, even in a child who has both. ADHD, a disorder known for inattentiveness, impulsivity, and hyperactivity, begins by age 6 and is characterized by acting before thinking, not by ritualizing in response to obsessions. Confusing these two is a good reason to seek out expert advice.

• *Some kids have OCD and something else.* Speaking of ADHD, another thing we know about kids with OCD is that some have this problem and no other mental disorders, whereas others have more than one illness. The other conditions that we see most often in children and teens with OCD are tic disorders, anxiety disorders, ADHD, and learning disorders. Some kids with OCD also suffer from depression, but more often than not depression is secondary to OCD and goes away all by itself when OCD is successfully treated.

• The program we offer in this book for helping kids with OCD is most effective for those diagnosed with OCD without a lot of other problems. That doesn't mean it can't be combined with other treatments for any additional conditions, but it does mean that a child who has other mental disorders or other problems might need an experienced therapist and a medical doctor who understands the issues that are involved in combining medications.

3

What Causes OCD?

"WHY IS THIS HAPPENING TO US?" is one of the most persistent, frustrating questions for families wrestling with OCD. Changes in a child's behavior can be extremely frightening for parents, and relentless obsessive thoughts and rituals can be very disturbing for the children who have them. Many families hold out hope that these OCD symptoms are just normal worries blown out of proportion and that giving a little extra attention to the child will shrink the problem back to normal proportions. As Chapter 2 explained, however, obsessions aren't just normal worries exaggerated. Unfortunately, before you knew that, you may have believed it was your fault that OCD was still around: You were doing something wrong, you were not doing something you should be doing, or maybe there was something wrong with your family life.

For years, the mental health profession mistakenly encouraged kids and families in such beliefs, even though addressing relationship issues made no difference in OCD symptoms. Scientists now know (and you do too if you read Chapters 1 and 2) that OCD is a neurological illness, a disorder located in the brain. Knowing this fact has helped many families deal with OCD in a more productive way, because, as an illness, OCD can be treated.

This chapter provides an outline of the neurobiology of OCD—what we know about brain structure and function in OCD—so that you can clearly label it a medical illness and get an idea of why cognitive-behavior therapy (CBT) can return your child's brain toward normal function. You'll also learn how children sometimes develop this brain disorder, but don't spend too much time worrying about how it all started. Just as spending a lot of time trying to figure out what triggers a particular obsession at a particular time doesn't get you anywhere, it's not very productive to try to determine how your child ended up with OCD. That's not generally the path to eliminating OCD from your child's life. Changing the behavior that keeps it going *is*.

Biology Is *Not* Destiny

Understanding how brain functions and structures differ in OCD has helped scientists arrive at treatments that can stop or reduce the symptoms of the illness we call OCD. (It has also helped them confirm that these treatments work, via neuroimaging techniques that show visible changes in the brain following treatment.) As you'll read in Chapter 4, medication is one of those treatments. Unfortunately, medication usually works only as long as kids keep taking it, and it doesn't work as well as CBT. The kind of CBT put to work in Part II of this book is more effective than medications and, if you take medications, may help you get off them. These proven methods we describe take advantage of the brain's most miraculous capacity: to learn. Using them, your child can retrain her brain's faulty stop signal so that the circuits involved in OCD stop hiccupping and don't start up again when medication is withdrawn.

For now, think of CBT and medications for OCD as the difference between doing physical therapy after spraining your ankle (like CBT) and just wearing an air cast (like medications). The therapy gives the joint lasting protection by strengthening the muscles that support your ankle. The air cast does the same while you wear it, but if you take it off, your ankle is vulnerable again. So it is with CBT and medications.

Biology does not have to be destiny in the case of OCD, thanks to the brain's capacity for learning. Kids can learn to play soccer, read, use a computer, and do other things that take some practice. Each one of these acquired skills reflects learning-induced changes in the brain. Likewise, we forget skills we don't use. Forgetting reflects changes in the brain, which doesn't waste resources on keeping up with things that have little or no useful purpose. Put simply, your brain is set up to reinforce what is used and to dump what isn't used.

What does this mean for OCD? As we explain later, the mental hiccups of OCD reflect a broken stop signal for certain kinds of automatic thoughts. Once it gets going, OCD is "overlearned," meaning that your child's brain has a lot of practice at OCD. Although OCD affects only a small segment of brain function relative to the rest of your child's perfectly good brain, the repetition of those hiccups causes big-time trouble. This doesn't mean that your child wants to think about OCD; it is just

WHAT TO SAY TO YOUR CHILD ABOUT OCD

"Picture what it would be like to ride your bike with the brakes broken. When you tried to put on the brakes, the bike would keep going: crash! But it wouldn't be because you were riding the bike wrong. It would be because a part of the bike wasn't working properly. That's what OCD is like: Those thoughts don't keep going because you're not a good kid; you are. There's something physically wrong with a stop signal for bad thoughts in a tiny and very specific part of the brain. The rest of your brain works fine, and you're no more crazy than I am. The good news is that, just like you can fix bike brakes, you can repair this hiccupping stop signal by changing your relationship to OCD, and when you do, the hiccups will stop."

that OCD is a really persistent mental hiccup. Your child works very hard at trying to get rid of OCD thoughts and to resist doing rituals, but he isn't very skillful at it. In fact, much of what he's doing now ends up giving OCD more power, with the results that the brain continues to practice OCD. To

WHAT TO SAY TO YOUR CHILD ABOUT OCD

"Your brain has gotten really good at OCD. The circuits in the brain that do OCD are strong, like they've been lifting weights, with all that practice doing what OCD wants. That's because your brain's stop signal isn't working right, not because you like it that way: OCD just keeps repeating itself, and the longer this goes on, the harder it is to get it to stop. We need to make a real effort to retrain that stop signal in your brain, so that OCD will quit hiccuping. That's what we're going to do with this program."

fix the broken stop signal and redirect the brain toward fun stuff, kids and teens with OCD need something skillful to *do* differently in response to OCD, which, of course, is why we put together the program in this book. We say: "OCD is not you, but you can do something about OCD!"

WHAT TO SAY TO YOUR CHILD ABOUT OCD

"You know Aaron, who hurt his knee playing soccer? He had to take Motrin and go see the physical therapist. Or, how about Stacey, who has diabetes and has to take shots and watch what she eats? Well, what we're going to do is like what the physical therapist did with Aaron or the nutritionist did with Stacey. We're going to help your brain stop hiccupping by teaching you some very specific things to do, just like Aaron had to do with his knee. It'll be a lot of work, but boy, will it feel good not to hurt anymore!"

While you learn how to deal with OCD skillfully, it is important to treat the child with OCD with a lot of kindness, because kids with OCD really can't yet willfully suppress obsessions and resist rituals most of the time. OCD is a disorder of brain circuits, not good or bad behavior. Understanding something about the brain circuitry involved

will help you all deal with rituals with compassion while your child is learning the skills to talk back to OCD. But, especially at times of particular stress, you may find the simpler metaphors that we've been using for OCD's maneuverings even more useful, because they're easier to call to mind quickly on command.

A Brief Review of What *Doesn't* Cause OCD

Although OCD seems to have been with us for thousands of years, the symptoms of obsessions and compulsions have been misunderstood and therefore wrongly diagnosed and poorly treated until very recently. Just so that you understand how firmly rooted in science our current understanding of the disorder is, here's a rundown of what we no longer believe:

Believe it or not, hundreds of years ago OCD was thought to be the result of demonic possession, to be cured by some type of exorcism or by repenting one's sins. Needless to say, that view of OCD not only prevented the development of effective treatments but also hurt many people terribly by saying that they were right to believe their obsessive thoughts were evil and that they were, too. Aren't we lucky to be living in the 21st century?

That view of OCD changed during the early 20th century thanks to Sigmund Freud and many family therapists. Freud attributed OCD to unconscious conflicts that started during toilet training and popped up later in life as obsessions and compulsions. Even though Freud himself wasn't entirely satisfied with this explanation and thought biological causes should be investigated, for decades people with OCD underwent lengthy psychoanalysis in a futile attempt to dredge up some key from the recesses of early childhood that would explain OCD. Well, that explanation didn't hold up either, and we now know that psychodynamic "play therapy" approaches to OCD don't reflect reality and don't work.

Family therapists, rather than claiming that the problem lay in the unconscious, speculated that OCD served a function in the family. In some family therapy circles, for example, it was common to claim that a child unconsciously volunteered to have OCD in order to distract from the parents' problems in their marriage and so to keep the family together. Not unexpectedly, such views often did more harm than good, because when OCD got worse with ineffective treatment, everybody ended up even angrier at each other than they were at the beginning. The plain truth is that therapies that are aimed at relationship issues or uncovering unconscious conflicts don't work for OCD. Nobody volunteers to have OCD, and there's nothing "back there" that needs uncovering—OCD itself is the problem.

Over the last 10 to 15 years, scientists in search of an external cause for OCD turned their focus to how OCD develops. They came up with the idea that OCD starts with a child having a very unpleasant experience with some normally unharmful thought or event—say, getting sick with the stomach flu on a field trip with lots of other kids also vomiting all over the bus. This experience would then lead the child to either avoid the same event in the future or to perform some ritual, such as washing her hands a lot, as a type of protective superstition. Pretty soon the superstition would spiral out of control, and before she knew it the child was washing for 3 or 4 hours a day.

By zeroing in on how thoughts and behaviors work together in OCD, this view contributed to the effective treatments we have today. But it didn't explain why some of us shrug off a bad thought or experience and others end up trapped by the obsessions and compulsions of OCD. More important, most people who have OCD cannot point to a specific event that triggered it. OCD usually begins insidiously, with just a few "bad" thoughts and a little more washing than usual until, after a while, it takes on a life of its own, and OCD mushrooms into view. In a few kids, mostly younger ones with an infectious form of OCD related to rheumatic fever (more on this later), the disorder begins like an explosion. Besides, whichever way it started, there's not much point in rummaging around in the past. When you're sick, you need a treatment aimed at your illness in the present so you can get rid of it now and for the future.

Scientists thought they had found the root cause when they discovered 25 years ago that medications such as clomipramine (brand name Anafranil) ease the symptoms of OCD. Clomipramine and other drugs like it ensure that there is enough of the chemical serotonin in certain areas of the brain, including the one that contains the broken OCD stop signal. The fact that these medications reduced obsessions and compulsions implied pretty strongly that OCD might be associated with low serotonin levels in the part of the brain that mediates the symptoms of OCD. Although we now know that low serotonin levels are one aspect of OCD, low serotonin is far from a complete explanation for OCD, and merely boosting brain serotonin is not enough for most patients to get well. (That is, as mentioned a little earlier, medication that boosts serotonin doesn't "cure" OCD.)

Although the scientific community is still a long way from fully understanding what causes OCD—in either children or adults—our knowledge has grown by leaps and bounds over the past 10 to 15 years, thanks to great strides in understanding the neurobiology of the disorder and what we've learned from implementing successful new treatments and studying their effects on the brain. We are now sure that OCD is a neuropsychiatric illness—a singular irregularity in brain function that is creating a very specific glitch in the child's thinking, feelings, and behavior.

How OCD Uses the Brain to Produce Obsessions and Compulsions

The brain is made up of many structures and circuits, all interconnected in a complicated web of loops and relays that we have just begun to understand. We call these circuits *neural networks*, and it is these networks that process information related to thoughts, feelings, and behaviors. For example, there are specific areas of the brain that handle attention, memory, and fears, and these areas talk to each other along well-defined pathways. In kids with OCD, these neural networks do their jobs properly most of the time. As you'll see, it is just one small bit that isn't working properly in OCD.

Some of these circuits, such as those involving the thinking mind, are unique to humans. Others, including those involving many of the more primitive fears typical of OCD—such as fears of harm to others, disgust, and the need for cleanliness—are common in at least nonhuman primates if not in all mammals. When scientists thought about the symptoms typically experienced in OCD, they categorized them as more complex than panic disorder, which is characterized in many patients by suffocation anxiety, and less complex than fears in generalized anxiety disorder, which involves excessive worry about real-life circumstances. Because neuroscientists already knew a lot about where fears of varying complexity and sophistication are regulated in the brain, they then were able to zero in on an older part of the brain that sits right behind the eye called the orbital frontal cortex as probably the site of the circuits that are hiccupping in OCD.

With the help of neuroimaging technologies (techniques that "take pictures" of the brain and its functioning), scientists exploring this part of the brain were ultimately able to see that people with OCD have a problem in the circuits that link an area of the brain called the *striatum* (where the faulty stop signal is located) via a brain relay center, the thalamus, to the orbital frontal cortex (where the fears are located).

Family Ties

Although the genes have yet to be identified, research also has shown clearly that OCD has a genetic basis. Early studies of OCD also showed that about 20% of kids with OCD had a family member with the disorder. Other family members had Tourette syndrome (TS), a disorder in which odd sensory feelings produce even odder movements, such as eye blinking, grimacing, or shoulder shrugging. These are called *tics*. A child with full TS also has vocal tics, such as throat clearing or other odd noises. We know that people with OCD have an increased rate of tic disorders and that those with tic disorders have an increased rate of OCD, which suggests

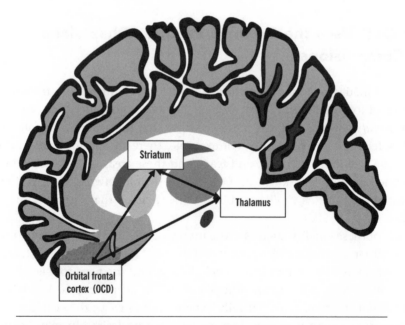

The cortical–thalamic–striatal–cortical circuit in OCD. Neuroimaging studies show abnormalities in these circuits when someone has active OCD and a return to normal when the person has had either cognitive-behavioral or drug treatment.

some kind of connection between these two illnesses. We also have evidence that first-degree relatives (siblings, parents, or children) of those with either OCD or TS show an increased rate of both tic disorders and OCD. When tics and OCD run in families, boys are more likely to have tics and girls are more likely to have OCD. What is really interesting is that the "flavor" or subtype of OCD (see Chapter 2) that a child has isn't inherited: Mom may have checking rituals where her son has washing rituals, for example.

All of these connections made scientists theorize that OCD and tic disorders are related genetic disorders—that they may in fact represent different expressions of the same gene(s) in some cases, though the specific genes involved have yet to be found. Just as important, both OCD and tic disorders involve faulty stop signals in the striatum, though the target symptom area differs: the orbitofrontal cortex in OCD and the sensory motor cortex, motor cortex, and supplementary motor area in tic disorders.

Strep Throat and OCD

Another fascinating discovery reinforced our understanding of the brain structures and circuits involved in OCD, and it also gave us an idea of one route by which kids might develop the disorder. Some younger children (preschool to early elementary school age), it turns out, seem to get OCD or tics or both after an infection with Group A beta hemolytic streptococcal infection (GABHS), what most of us know as "strep throat." Researchers at the National Institute of Mental Health (NIMH) call this "pediatric autoimmune neuropsychiatric disorder associated with strep (PANDAS)." PANDAS is related to rheumatic fever, a rare outcome of strep infection that causes problems with the heart and an inflammatory kind of arthritis. OCD symptoms are common in children with another form of rheumatic fever called Sydenham's chorea. In Sydenham's chorea, patients make movements that look a lot like the complex tics seen in TS. Like rheumatic heart disease or arthritis, Sydenham's is believed to involve inflammation of the area of the brain that controls the OCD stop signal. This inflammation is caused by an immune reaction to the cell wall of the streptococcal bacteria.

Because the strep bacteria has evolved to camouflage itself by coming to look like the body, the immune system gets confused and attacks the body itself—the heart (causing rheumatic carditis), the joints (causing rheumatic arthritis), or the striatum (causing Sydenham's chorea, OCD, and tics).

WHAT TO SAY TO YOUR CHILD ABOUT OCD

"Sometimes people in the same family have OCD or another type of illness related to OCD. Just as diabetes or arthritis or other diseases run in families, OCD seems to do so as well. It would be better if this weren't so, but everyone has something that they're vulnerable to. We can't choose the genetic hand we're dealt. The trick is to respond to it skillfully, and the good news is that OCD is actually easier to treat than many other medical problems."

These are called *autoimmune disorders*: *auto* because the body gets confused and attacks itself and *immune* because it does so using procedures that fight off foreign invaders, such as bacteria or viruses. We now think that a small proportion of early childhood OCD that comes on explosively or gets worse after a bout of strep throat involves an autoimmune mechanism. This implies that treatments for rheumatic fever, including prescribing antibiotics or clearing the bloodstream of antineuronal antibodies, may be of benefit to some children with clearly documented PANDAS. However, this subject is still actively being researched, so it does not yet make sense to treat children and teenagers who have OCD with rheumatic fever treatments. We simply treat strep throat when it is present and use the other treatments we have to treat OCD.

Brain Hiccups: The Brain Structure and Activity Behind OCD

We have a lot of evidence that the cause of OCD is in fact localized to a circuit that connects the orbital frontal cortex, where complex emotions are located, and the striatum, where the traffic lights controlling habitual behaviors are found. Some of it we've already mentioned, like PANDAS. But we also often see symptoms that resemble OCD in people who have suffered injuries and disorders to the striatum and orbital frontal cortex. Brain infections, head injury, epileptic seizures, and brain tumors located in or around the OCD circuitry can produce the illness.

These facts strongly suggest that this area of the brain plays a key role in the symptoms of OCD. Until 20 years ago, however, researchers were limited to a lot of guesswork, because they simply didn't have a way to see what went on inside the brain. Now we have several different brain-scanning technologies that can provide pictures that allow us to compare the structures and activity of the brains of people with a specific illness such as OCD to those of people without the illness. We can also look at how the brain works (or, better said, doesn't work) before and after it responds to treatment. The new information this has provided about how certain illnesses work, what might cause them, and how to treat them is mind boggling.

In the case of OCD, PET (positron emission tomography) scans in particular have supplied a big piece of evidence that OCD is so firmly rooted in biology that many scientists today have suggested OCD may rightly be considered a neurological disease rather than a psychiatric disorder. (But then again, research increasingly indicates that psychiatry and neurology will come together as we learn more about what the brain does or doesn't do in neuropsychiatric illnesses of all kinds.) PET scans work by detecting a small amount of radiation that has been added to a sugar molecule injected into a person's bloodstream as that sugar molecule travels to the brain. The most common sugar is glucose, a simple sugar that provides the fuel on which the brain runs. Because sugar is food for the brain cells, observing where sugar is used in the brain tells scientists how much activity is going on in various parts of the brain.

Scientists have done PET scans like this on people with OCD and then compared them with those of people without OCD. These comparisons have shown that people with OCD have an overactive orbital frontal cortex and caudate nucleus. As a result, researchers now believe that the broken stop signal at work in OCD resides in an essential pathway in the brain that involves the three anatomical brain regions mentioned earlier, the orbital frontal cortex, the striatum (especially the caudate nucleus), and the thalamus. The orbital frontal cortex, which is located just behind the eyeball, is the part of the brain that notices when something isn't quite right. The orbital frontal cortex then works with other structures to process this information and to develop a plan of action that is appropriate to the situation. For example, if the orbital frontal cortex registers that there is something dirty or disgusting nearby, it sends a "worry" signal to the thalamus via the striatum. The thalamus then relays this signal to other areas of the brain and feeds relevant information back to the orbital frontal cortex. The caudate nucleus lies between the orbital frontal cortex and the thalamus and regulates signals sent between them, forming a loop or circuit that handles complex worries about such things as contamination, harm to others, moral thinking, and the need for certainty.

Everyone has troublesome thoughts that sometimes just arise spontaneously and sometimes are triggered by something in the environment. When the circuit linking the orbital frontal cortex to the thalamus and back again is working properly, the caudate nucleus acts like the brake pedal on a car, suppressing the worry signal sent by the orbital frontal cortex to the thalamus. In short, the caudate nucleus acts as a stop signal to prevent senseless worries from using up brain processing time. In OCD, the stop signal in the caudate nucleus is thought to be damaged, so it cannot suppress signals from the orbital frontal cortex. The thalamus is allowed to become overexcited, and—boom—the whole circuit gets the hiccups. The person then responds to these thoughts and bad feelings by doing the appropriate thing, but because the circuit won't turn off, what would be ordinary washing in response to a contamination worry turns into compulsive ritualizing. Over time, the circuit becomes overlearned, so it hiccups even without a triggering stimulus, and OCD is the result.

When OCD starts hiccupping, it sets off alarms that cause the child to pay more attention, feel anxious, or experience other negative emotions and that make the child vulnerable to getting lost in thoughts about and within the experience that we call an attack of OCD. This explains why it's so hard for your child to resist performing rituals—and why, as you'll see, our approach to treatment works precisely because it teaches your child how to retrain these basic brain processes by thinking about the obsessions differently and by refraining from doing rituals.

Another valuable scanning device, called MRI (magnetic resonance imaging), uses a powerful magnet to produce very detailed pictures of brain structures. MRI has proven particularly useful with kids, as research with PET can't ethically be done in children with OCD because of the radiation exposure. MRI can take pictures of brain structures to check on their size and location (so-called volumetric MRI). It can also produce images of the brain at work—the so-called functional magnetic resonance imaging, or fMRI. And one form of MRI, called magnetic resonance spectroscopy (or MRS), can even show the neurotransmitters at work in the brain structures that may be involved in illnesses such as OCD. All three types of MRI (volumetric, functional, and MRS) have been applied to OCD in children and adolescents. The take-home message is that overactive circuits that link the striatum, particularly the caudate nucleus, the thalamus, and the orbital frontal cortex seem to be involved in OCD in children and adolescents, just as they are in adults. Although we have much to learn, it's another bit of evidence that brain irregularities are at the root of OCD (and that serotonin levels are not the whole story about what causes the disorder).

David Rosenberg and Andrew Gilbert showed, using volumetric MRI, that the thalamus was larger in children with OCD than in normal children. Even more significantly, they then went on to show that the size of the thalamus returned to normal after 12 weeks of treatment with medication and that this decrease was directly related to improvement in OCD.

Other studies have been showing for quite some time that activity in the essential orbital frontal cortex–striatum–thalamus pathway becomes normal in people with OCD once they are treated with either medication or cognitive behavioral therapy like the program your child will learn in this book. The first studies of this type, which were done by Jeff Schwartz and Lew Baxter at UCLA in the early 1990s, used PET scanning in adults to show that either medication or CBT could return OCD circuits to normal in patients who responded positively to treatment.

Dr. Rosenberg's group has preliminary data showing that the same thing happens in children and adolescents. These scientists have shown that fast-acting neurotransmission in the head of the caudate nucleus seems to slow down as these hiccupping circuits return to normal—less so with CBT than with medications—whereas choline, another neurotransmitter localized to the thalamus, may be returning toward normal in children treated with CBT. What is really exciting is that preliminary data suggests that this is happening by a direct effect of medication and by an indirect effect—top-down regulation of the thalamus by the prefrontal or thinking cortex—with CBT. (As you'll learn in Chapter 4, it's the CBT, which engages the brain mechanisms involved with learning, that also seems to protect kids against relapse; this effect implies that CBT produces the more lasting effects.)

WHAT TO SAY TO YOUR CHILD ABOUT OCD

"It's good to know that you don't have OCD because of something you—or we—are doing wrong. But if OCD has something to do with your genes, you might be worried that you can't do anything about it, any more than you can change the brown eyes you got from Dad or the great singing voice you got from Grandma. Luckily, your brain is smart enough to get around vulnerabilities your genes may be creating. Right now doctors don't know how to 'fix' genes, but certain types of medication can slow down those nagging thoughts, and the steps in this book can help your brain learn to ignore OCD so that the brain circuits that do OCD can quiet down."

Another Piece of the Neurological Puzzle: The Chemical Messengers

We know that the neural circuits that connect the orbital frontal cortex, the striatum, and the thalamus are involved in causing OCD because scans have shown greater activity and different structure in those areas compared with people without OCD. But we also know that serotonin reuptake inhibitors reduce obsessions and compulsions in people with OCD. So maybe the specific cause of OCD is related to how serotonin regulates this circuit. As a matter of fact, we do think that problems with serotonin are involved in the overactivity in the orbital frontal cortex and striatum. But we really don't know enough about how the brain works to say that serotonin levels are solely responsible. For one thing, we don't know *why* they seem to be low. For another, we don't know what, if anything, serotonin levels have to do with the structural differences that we see in the brains of people with OCD.

The picture below depicts a typical serotonin synapse. Nerve cells carry messages from one neuron to the next. Neurons meet each other at the synapse, which is why the junction between two neurons is called the synaptic space or cleft. Referring to where they sit relative to the synaptic space, the front neuron is called the presynaptic neuron and the next neuron in line is called the postsynaptic neuron. When the presynaptic neuron wants to tell the postsynaptic neuron to fire, it releases serotonin into the synapse. Serotonin then travels (diffuses) over to the postsynaptic neuron, where it binds to a specific receptor, which initiates the firing mechanism. To turn the postsynaptic receptor off—the switch would be useless

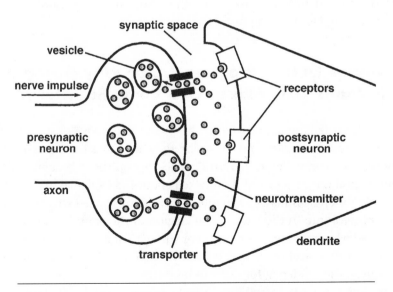

Typical serotonin synapse.

without an off mechanism, too—serotonin is reabsorbed into the presynaptic neuron. This is the so-called serotonin reuptake site. The serotonin transporter acts like a conveyer belt to pull serotonin back into the presynaptic neuron, where it can be repackaged. The transporter mechanism is not only the off switch but also the brain's recycling mechanism for serotonin.

Serotonin reuptake inhibitors (SRIs) interfere with the process by which serotonin is reabsorbed into the presynaptic neuron by blocking reuptake of serotonin by the serotonin transporter. In turn, this makes it more likely that the postsynaptic neuron will stay active. When serotonin is low in the synapses, the person may suffer depression, anxiety, mood swings, or, as it turns out, OCD. Serotonin is in short supply in a child with OCD as compared with a "control" child (one without OCD). By poisoning the serotonin transporter, SRIs strengthen serotonin's messages, normalizing these regulatory functions in people who have too little synaptic serotonin. More serotonin in the head of the caudate, not incidentally, coincides with a decrease in OCD symptoms.

Why should changing levels of serotonin make a difference? Perhaps because serotonin controls the levels of another neurotransmitter called glutamate, which is what carries "fast" messages in the brain. We have known for a long time that it takes weeks for the SRI to make a difference in OCD, so it can't be just a matter of turning off a stuck "on" switch. Rather, the SRI must be changing the tendency of the circuit to fire off by modifying fast glutaminergic neural activity, which is just what Dr. Rosenberg has discovered using MRS. He measured the levels of glutamate before and after treatment with an SRI in a child with OCD. Glutamate levels were substantially reduced in the head of the caudate, suggesting that the SRI "turns down" fast-acting neurotransmission in the "stop signal" region of the brain, thereby improving OCD symptoms.

What Causes OCD to Progress . . . or Why Giving It What It Wants Only Makes OCD Come Back for More

So far we've been talking about what makes people with OCD react differently to common situations than other people—why they are subject to obsessive thoughts and why they are compelled to perform rituals to stop those thoughts. We started with neurological differences and then talked about the evidence that the tendency to have those differences may be inherited. We then discussed why we think faulty regulation of serotonin in the "stop signal" region of the brain has something to do with OCD and why treatment with an SRI or with CBT may help some people. There is, however, another facet of OCD that makes life so hard for the families that OCD strikes, namely, the tendency for OCD to be progressive.

To see how this looks in real life, consider a boy whose OCD makes him check locks. Billy started out checking the lock once, but before long he was checking for hours and involving his dad in the ritual. OCD also got Billy to check other doors in the house. Once a child with OCD yields to the illness and starts to check repeatedly, those cues get locked into the brain, and the circuits that do OCD get stronger and stronger as the triggers for obsessions are followed by more and more rituals. Billy's brain has overlearned to check locks when the idea that doors might be unlocked and expose the family to danger comes up. It has overlearned the idea that the doors might be unlocked in the first place.

The important point here is that eliminating compulsions seems to be key to preventing OCD from getting worse and then eliminating it entirely from a child's life. When a child resists performing rituals, the triggers for OCD are no longer locked in, which means that the obsessions will not arise and repeat themselves and the child won't experience the need to do rituals. This means that on a neurological level the key to curing OCD lies in behaviorally reinforcing the brain's "stop signal," which in turn basically means teaching Billy how not to do what OCD tells him to do. This means that Billy needs to relearn how to think about OCD and then how to behave skillfully in relation to OCD so that his brain can return to normal functioning. Working with Dr. Rosenberg, we have been using MRS to gather the information that shows how the tools we present in this book can rehabilitate the stop signal in the brain so that OCD will be turned off rather than on. Although this work is still in the very preliminary stages, we are hopeful that work with children will replicate work by Drs. Baxter and Schwartz in showing that CBT with kids, as well as with adults, returns brain function to normal.

Back to the Beginning

Though, of course, the brain is enormously more complicated than what we've presented in this chapter, the diagram on the following page summarizes what we've learned about OCD as a medical illness. OCD symptoms arise on a circuit that connects the orbital frontal cortex (symptom location) to the striatum (stop signal). When the stop signal fails, the circuit hiccups. SRIs reinforce the stop signal by slowing down fast neurotransmission in the striatum. CBT works by retraining the stop signal in two ways. First, by downward regulation from the frontal "thinking" cortex and probably by recruiting normal stop signal circuits to help out, CBT overrides the urge to do rituals, which in turn causes the striatum to slow down from lack of exercise. Second, CBT teaches the frontal "thinking" cortex to talk directly to the orbital frontal cortex, telling it to "quiet down—there's nothing to worry about." In short, CBT blocks the tendency of OCD to overpower voluntary frontal cortical control of normal thinking and behavior. The medication bolsters control of inhibition at the level of the striatum (from the bottom up), while the program in this book acts to stop obsessions and compulsions "from the top down."

This brings us full circle. We know that the mind fills up with senseless thoughts (obsessions) that use up a lot of the child's brain resources in getting upset (complex emotions) and that these emotions in turn drive a set of excessive behav-

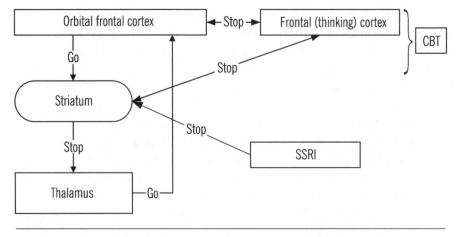

The brain circuit involved in OCD symptoms.

iors designed to make the child feel better (compulsions). We know the location of the brain structures that play a role in these phenomena, and we can watch them at work in normal life and in disease. We know that our treatments work to return these structures toward normal functioning, so that information is processed normally in the brain. Most important, we know that biology really doesn't have to be destiny. The mind is not just what the brain does. You are not the same thing as your brain, any more than the idea of time is the same thing as the gears in a watch. By changing your relationship to OCD, you can make a difference. With the proven CBT strategies outlined in this book, your son or daughter has a very good chance of returning his or her brain toward normal and, in doing so, to get rid of OCD and keep it gone. Chapter 4 explains more about the treatments that we know help show OCD the door.

4

How Is OCD Treated?

IF YOUR FAMILY HAS BEEN FIGHTING a losing battle with obsessions and compulsions, a diagnosis of OCD and the promise of effective treatment can be the turning point you've been looking for. Now that you know what's wrong, you can take advantage of treatments that return the great majority of kids and teens to their normal daily lives. Playing soccer is always better than going to the doctor.

The latest studies show that the program we offer in Part II can eliminate OCD from the lives of about half of the kids who stick with the therapy for 3 months. Even those who still have some symptoms will be a lot better. Medication reduces OCD symptoms significantly too, for those who need the extra boost, but it isn't as good by itself as the program in this book. Although more research is necessary, we also believe that when medication is the only treatment and then is discontinued, kids are much more likely to relapse than they are when they've completed CBT before stopping medication.

For this reason, and so that you'll have a good foundation of knowledge to start the program, this chapter concentrates on explaining the type of CBT that we now know is effective even without medication for kids who have mild to moderate OCD. Kids who have more severe OCD can benefit too, but they may need medication in addition, at least at the beginning of treatment. The last sections of this chapter discuss what you need to know about the medications currently used to treat OCD in children and teenagers.

What Is CBT?

We've made a lot of references to cognitive-behavioral therapy, or CBT, in this book without getting into what it is. To put it simply, CBT is a combination of cognitive therapy and behavior therapy.

In behavior therapy—the BT in CBT—people are shown how to change thoughts and feelings that are causing them trouble by first changing their behavior. Many different types of behavior therapy (and CBT) have been developed by psychologists to treat different problems. They have been proven effective for depression, anxiety, and bipolar disorder, among many other psychiatric disorders. The form that is so effective with OCD that it has become part of the treatment of choice for the illness is called "exposure and response prevention," or EX/RP (you may also see this abbreviated as ERP or E/RP). Later in this chapter we explain how EX/RP works for kids, teens, and adults with OCD.

Cognitive therapy—the C in CBT—focuses on what people are thinking, helping them challenge unhelpful thoughts that are making them feel bad and behave in ways that aren't serving them well. Cognitive therapy might help someone examine and replace inaccurate beliefs (such as a depressed person's belief that he's powerless or the exaggerated sense that kids with OCD often have that they are responsible for the welfare of loved ones). For kids with OCD, one of the most important parts of cognitive therapy is changing their view of their relationship to OCD. Through what you've read so far in this book, both you and your child have already received a little cognitive therapy, as you have been helped to understand the need to treat OCD as an illness, something separate from the child. As you'll see, it's just as important for you to absorb that message as it is for your child, because it undergirds your entire role in the program that follows.

Choosing the Best Treatment for the Child or Teen

Both CBT and medication have been proven effective (in different ways and to different degrees) for kids and teens with OCD, but which children get which kinds of treatment, and how are those decisions made? Ideally, your child's doctor, the child, and you—often, in fact, the whole family—will team up to figure out the best possible treatment plan for your son or daughter. The plan may call for medications or CBT or both, depending on a variety of factors related to the illness and to the family's preferences for treatment, along with the doctor's. It may include other types of therapy, such as family therapy (if your family is undergoing a lot of battles that get in the way of using CBT on your own) or less formal support groups that can help everyone profit from the experience of other kids or adults who've had OCD. *It should not include unproven treatments such as play therapy, family therapies that see OCD as a symptom of family conflict, or psychoanalysis or medications other than serotonin reuptake inhibitors (SRIs).* Your child's treatment may be closely supervised by a physician and/or a therapist or carried out largely through self-help. The initial plan may work like a charm, or it may require some trial and error to become as effective as it can be.

A successful treatment plan will take into account the child's exact diagnosis and a number of other factors that are best determined by the doctor, such as the characteristics of the illness (e.g., severity or type of symptoms) or the presence of other mental disorders (such as ADHD or depression) that might call for a more complex combination of treatments. If, for example, your child is also suffering from depression, you and the doctor might choose CBT for OCD, plus a selective serotonin reuptake inhibitor (SSRI) for depression. This would be like physical therapy for a blown-out knee plus Motrin for general relief of arthritis symptoms. Or you might choose just CBT for OCD, expecting that reducing trouble from OCD will also reduce the depression. Toss ADHD into the mix and the drug treatment now grows to include a psychostimulant, such as Ritalin, and the psychosocial intervention may need to include parent training. In making recommendations in these areas, family input is super important, not only because you know the child with OCD best but also because, if you don't all understand and sign on to the treatment plan, it won't get done, and your child will be much less likely to get well again.

Although families don't cause OCD, families are important! Your doctor will want to understand the family context in which OCD occurs and the treatment will take place. To make the best recommendations for treatment, the doctor needs to understand how the family generally operates, what the pace of family life is like, and how the family members interact. As you know, family members are often (but not always) tangled up in OCD too, so any treatment that is to be effective has to consider all of you. The doctor's goal in treatment should be to help you ally with each other to help defeat OCD and in so doing to capitalize on what everyone in the family is already doing well and what their strengths, hopes, and wishes are. To determine this, when I meet a family one of my first tasks is to learn about the child's relationship with herself concerning OCD and about how OCD has influenced the parents' relationship with the child. My goal is not to figure out what caused OCD but rather to understand how OCD affects the child and how everyone in the family feels and acts in relation to OCD. Hearing people's stories helps me understand how the family can better work together to fight OCD.

What Does It Take to Make Treatment a Success?

Though we are rightly attracted to the wonders of medical technology, medicine has always been and remains as much a story of the heart as of the body. While we will teach you to treat OCD impersonally—it is an illness, not a part of who one is as a person—it matters that you have OCD. Because learning new ways of working skillfully with OCD involves changing your own story about the illness, your family's willingness to turn the page and write a new story may matter more to treatment outcome than whether, say, your child is a teenager or a boy or what your family's social or economic status is. We call this willingness to think about OCD differently "readiness to change," and the more ready your child and your family are to change, the better your chances are of doing what you need to do to help the child with OCD get well again.

Everyone, we have discovered, starts out with the same chance—a very good one—of beating OCD. Add in various factors and the road gets rougher or smoother, but the final destination can still be a positive outcome. Calm, supportive families help, whereas overcritical, overinvolved families may unwittingly make OCD worse. Youngsters from well-adjusted families with good health insurance and knowledgeable doctors typically do better with any illness than those beset with more adversity in their personal lives. But even when adversity is present, a strong family–doctor–patient alliance can address it by working together to make sure the child gets the treatment needed.

Although other factors play a role, however, perhaps the biggest positive factor is access to a doctor who knows what OCD is and how to treat it. (For more information on finding a doctor who knows about OCD, as well as other sources of information, see the back of this book.) For a child who hasn't yet been diagnosed with OCD, getting a confirmed diagnosis is an important first step. After that, it's extremely beneficial to have a professional on hand to help as needed with the program in this book once you've decided to make it part of your child's treatment. But even if you don't have a doctor who specializes in CBT, your child and you can give it a try simply by following the directions in Part II. (See the Introduction for more specific advice for determining whether you're likely to succeed with the program as pure self-help rather than guided self-help—that is, with the assistance of a therapist.)

Expert Consensus Treatment Guidelines

To help doctors make decisions regarding the treatment of OCD, we have developed a set of expert guidelines for practitioners who have less experience in treating OCD to help them answer questions such as these:

- When should a doctor use CBT with children and adolescents with OCD?
- When should a doctor use drug therapy?
- Is there an advantage to combining CBT and drug therapy?
- When should a doctor change course in treatment?
- Once the patient is better, what should the doctor do?

The following guidelines are based on the expert survey on OCD, which you can read for yourself at *www.psychguides.com*. We've included only those pertinent to kids for whom it makes sense to use CBT and/or drug therapy. The full guidelines also tell us what the experts think is the best strategy for a child who has already tried a certain treatment regimen that hasn't worked well, how to handle stopping treatment, and how best to handle comorbidity (having more than one disorder). The following guidelines are backed up by our recent research, which clearly shows that CBT with or without medications is the key to getting well.

- For children who haven't reached puberty, CBT is the initial treatment of choice, whether the OCD is mild or more severe.
- For adolescents, CBT is the first treatment of choice when the OCD is mild;

when it is more severe, the first choice should be CBT, and then medications if the CBT isn't working well, or CBT plus an SSRI from the start.

- If the child or teen is too sick to start off with CBT—for example, the child has severe OCD plus severe depression—treatment probably should start with an SSRI. Once the edge is off OCD and depression is improved, which usually takes about 6 weeks, CBT for both OCD and depression should be started.

Severity will be determined by the doctor, using various rating scales such as the simple one at the back of this book and at the end of the kids' section of Chapter 5 (used throughout the program) and/or more detailed ones. If your doctor takes a radically different course from this one, be sure to ask why and think carefully about whether the doctor and the treatment are right for you and your child.

Thirteen-year-old Nathan feels like OCD is looking over his shoulder, glued to him like his shadow, every second of the day. Not only does OCD interfere with every part of his daily routine, from getting dressed to going to the bathroom to eating, but it's started to make it impossible for him to go to school. He just can't do anything on the same schedule as the other kids, can't concentrate on tests, and can't get most homework done. OCD has changed his life so thoroughly that Nathan has become depressed. The previously gregarious boy has started saying that he doesn't see any point in trying and that he "can't do anything right." He doesn't talk to his friends anymore or even get excited about the Knicks games, although he was once an avid basketball fan. Nathan's doctor started him on fluoxetine (Prozac). After about 3 weeks Nathan started to be able to do a few things without OCD hovering nearby, and his parents reported that he'd perked up for the first time in months. His doctor called the family together to talk about CBT, referred them to a local support group, and set up appointments to start the kind of therapy program presented in this book.

Madison had a lot of counting rituals that OCD had foisted on her. For the most part, she could keep them hidden while at school, by doing them in her head. But they were beginning to take up more and more time, and her grades were slipping as she got more and more "spacy" (the teacher's observation). By the time Maddie got home, she was so exhausted and stressed out from trying to keep OCD under control at school that she would dissolve in tears at the slightest hassle or start picking fights with her little sister. When her parents had her evaluated and she was diagnosed with moderate OCD, the family agreed to give CBT a try. A month into her therapy, Maddie's grades were beginning to pick up. A couple of months later she felt like OCD was gone except for an occasional urge to count things when she was really, really tired or nervous. Then she pulled out the tools her therapist had taught her and sent OCD on its way again.

Jorge was a really miserable 11-year-old struggling with what felt like constant harangues from OCD that he had caused his father's cancer and that he was going to make the rest of his family sick too, unless he followed very strict "rules" for washing himself and most of what he touched in the house. Jorge didn't have any problem with OCD at school, as long as he washed his hands for 10 minutes before getting on the bus to go home. He could keep it together when he needed to take his little brothers and sisters to the park or go to the store while his mom took his dad for chemotherapy. But when his doctor started a CBT program with Jorge, they quickly found that Jorge's guilt over the idea that he had made his father sick and would make his mother and siblings sick too, and his fear of being left alone with no family were so great that he couldn't bring himself to talk back to OCD. His therapist added sertraline (Zoloft) and put CBT on hold for a few weeks. When they tried again, Jorge was able to make progress and finished the CBT program in 3 months. Then his doctor gradually took him off the medication, reminding him of all the tools he had learned to use that would keep OCD away if it tried to interfere in Jorge's life again.

Amy, a 14-year-old with contamination fears and washing rituals, had seen lots of doctors for OCD. All of them gave her medicines, usually more than one. OCD just got worse and worse, and she gained a lot of weight. It was pretty clear to Amy and her mom that the SSRIs all helped a little and that nothing else gave much benefit, only nasty side effects. Worse, the doctors didn't seem to understand that Amy wanted to know what to do in response to OCD. She didn't just want another pill. When she found her way to our clinic, we stopped all her medications and began CBT. Within 3 months, she was much better, but not all the way better. It turned out that medication was helpful but only in combination with CBT. Her medication was restarted (at a lower dose to produce fewer side effects), and within 6 months Amy was completely well, had lost most of the weight she'd gained, and was trying out for the soccer team at her high school.

CBT, Medication, or Combination Treatment?

All the experts agree today that treatments that work for kids with OCD fall into two categories: medication management with an SRI and CBT. Other medications and other kinds of psychotherapy do not work for OCD. Studies have shown that medications reduce symptoms in a meaningful way after a couple of months in about two-thirds of children with OCD. But what isn't generally known is that only about one in five children treated with an SSRI alone will no longer have OCD. In contrast, research has shown that almost everyone treated with CBT using the procedures outlined in this book will experience at least some relief and that about 40% with CBT alone will no longer have OCD. Amazingly, over half of the children and adolescents treated with both CBT and an SSRI will no longer have OCD after 12 weeks.

In a landmark study funded by the National Institute of Mental Health and published in the *Journal of the American Medical Association,* we recently compared the responses of children and teenagers to the different types of treatment: placebo (sugar pill), sertraline (an SSRI), cognitive-behavioral therapy (CBT, the program in this book), and a combination of CBT and sertraline. As the graph below shows, children benefited overwhelmingly from either CBT alone or CBT plus sertraline. Hardly anyone got better with placebo (the sugar pill), and far fewer benefited from medication alone than from CBT.

In our clinic at Duke, where we treat lots of kids who have not responded to previous treatments, more than 90% of the kids with OCD who have gone through our program have either eliminated OCD from their lives or reduced it to a manageable problem.

It's not surprising that medications and CBT are effective in treating OCD, because the disorder is a medical illness and, as we've seen, both medications and behavioral changes are widely used and effective for most medical illnesses. What is surprising is that both CBT and medications seem to produce some of the same changes in the brain, returning the brain structures that are different in people with OCD to normal. As we discussed in Chapter 3, work by our group in collaboration

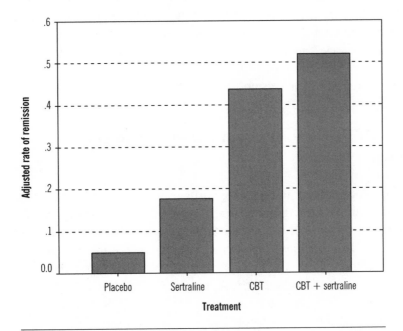

The POTS study showed that CBT and CBT plus sertraline (CBT + sertraline) were much more effective than either sertraline alone or a placebo (sugar pill).

"The medicine that some kids take to help them get rid of OCD is sort of like the volume knob on the TV. The medicine turns down the volume of obsessions and makes it easier to ignore OCD when it wants you to do its rituals. But you still need to make the decision about whether to go along with OCD in doing the rituals, and the program in this book will help you decide how and when not to do that. Pills don't make choices, people do, and this program will help us all make choices that will spell the end of OCD."

with David Rosenberg at Wayne State University in Detroit, Michigan, seems to suggest that CBT helps to calm down the overactive circuits that control OCD symptoms but by a different mechanism from that of the SSRIs. This, combined with the fact that the effects of CBT seem to last longer when treatment is discontinued, suggests that the treatments may target the brain in significantly different ways and that perhaps combining CBT and medication ought to enhance the effects of either treatment individually. For some kids, then, combining medications and CBT may deliver more improvement than either one alone, and that's exactly what we've found, as shown in the graph.

Why then isn't CBT plus an SSRI always the first choice for treating kids and teens? Simply because caution tells us that young people should not receive medications unless they are determined to be necessary. More on this subject is presented later in the chapter. The bottom line? Comparisons of treatment effectiveness, such as our previously described study, are important when making decisions about what type of treatment your child should get, but they're not the only things that should inform your choices. Your decision should also be based on an understanding of how CBT of the type laid out in this book works and of the pros and cons of the medications prescribed for kids and teens with OCD.

CBT for OCD: How Exposure and Response Prevention Works

EX/RP empowers children to do the opposite of what OCD tells them to do—that's why we call our program "talking back to OCD." When OCD says "avoid," we say "confront." That's the *exposure*. When OCD says "do rituals," we say "refrain from doing rituals." This is *response prevention*. Together, exposure and response prevention mean facing whatever triggers the child's obsessions and then resisting the compulsion to perform the usual ritual. This is not the same thing as "just stop it." The secret is in how EX/RP is done: slowly, under the child's control, beginning with the easy stuff that the child is already successfully resisting some of the time. The rest is off limits, meaning that you do the best you can without guilt or blaming. The child with OCD moves to more difficult exposures only once she has succeeded in resisting the compulsions that are the target of EX/RP.

Say your son's obsession is that he will make your family sick if he doesn't wash his hands 20 times before entering the kitchen and touching any food or dishes. He might start by trying to wash his hands only 15 times instead of 20 or by resisting washing his hands when touching only food that he's going to eat or by resisting washing his hands before entering the kitchen only once a day for the first week. All the time he's telling himself that OCD is just a brain hiccup and doesn't mean anything, nothing bad will happen, and that he can and must do this to get well again. The way we use EX/RP, the boy is in charge of the pace of his therapy so that he doesn't end up feeling so anxious or uncomfortable that he feels he can't do it.

What we believe happens in the mind over time spent using EX/RP is that the child (and his brain) begins to recognize more and more that the exposure did not produce the consequence he feared. Touching things in the kitchen, for example, did not make anyone in his family sick. The more he and his brain realize this, the less OCD is able to stick those obsessions into his head.

The first two cases of effective OCD treatment using EX/RP were reported as long ago as 1966, and since then we've known it is a remarkably effective treatment in adults. In fact, around 1980, evidence began to accumulate that behavior therapy and medications both worked to dampen OCD symptoms, with CBT perhaps working a bit better.

We don't have as long a history of or as much research with children, but evidence in its favor is constantly mounting. Children, however, often need to be motivated to participate in CBT in ways that pay attention to their age. For example, young children handle EX/RP best when it's turned into a game or a kind of contest. In Part II we'll give lots of ideas for modifying our program so that it matches up well with what your child needs to get motivated to do the CBT program.

Although exposure and response prevention (the behavioral therapy part of CBT) is the heart of the treatment, we have found over time that how children think and talk to themselves about OCD is very important in making a success of EX/RP. We call this the cognitive aspect of the treatment (the C in CBT). The goals of cognitive therapy, which may be more or less useful or necessary depending on the child and the nature of the child's OCD, are essentially to make the child feel capable of turning the tables on OCD—to make him feel like he can predict what will happen despite OCD's intrusions, control the situation, and produce a good outcome of the EX/RP tasks. Specifically, your child will learn how to:

- Talk to herself in a realistic and positive way about resisting OCD: "It'll be hard, but I know that I can do this."
- Confront goofy OCD thinking: "Even though OCD says I'll be to blame, I know that if something bad happens it's not my fault."
- Detach from OCD by cultivating a sense that OCD is impersonal: "OCD is just a brain hiccup and, kind of like the weather, it will pass, so I don't need to do anything except smile and practice being patient until it goes away on its own."

EX/RP is what makes the treatment of OCD go forward. More or less weight can be placed on the cognitive facet of the treatment, depending on the child's particular OCD symptoms. For example, a child with urge-driven "just so" rituals—in which things need to be evened up or balanced—might not use the tool for confronting goofy thinking, whereas cultivating the ability to watch OCD as though it is a passing cloud could be very important in making a success of response prevention.

The goal of CBT programs such as ours is to bring the child to the point at which obsessions rarely intrude on the child's day and at which, when they do, the child has a kit full of tools primed to deal with them before they lead to even more disruptive compulsions. Most children and teenagers can reach this point within a few short weeks if they are diligent about following the program.

How our program works is detailed in full in Chapter 5. But as a parent it's critical for you to know what your role will be, because your child will need a very specific type and degree of help from you to make the treatment a success.

Your Role in CBT

Whether you intend to or not, you may very well have found yourself "helping" your child complete OCD rituals. It's awfully hard not to help a child line up his shoes or to agree to wash all of his clothes over and over when he seems so distressed about his shoes being out of line or his clothes being "full of germs." Once you start helping in this way, it's hard to stop. *But in this program you'll have to, because the biggest pitfall for kids undertaking CBT is the tendency to bail out of exposure and yield to the compulsion to do a ritual. EX/RP can't succeed when a child bails out.* This doesn't mean that you'll need to become a tough taskmaster for your child to make sure he sticks with the program. On the contrary, you can't be *any* kind of taskmaster. For your child to really come to believe that obsessions are just brain hiccups and that rituals aren't necessary or helpful, he has to take charge of the program himself. But there are ways for you to participate that can support your child's efforts.

We've found that having a new script is the best way to ease yourself out of participating in the child's rituals. Instead of trying to talk your child out of performing a ritual or helping with it, you can learn to express empathy while gently encouraging your child to talk back to OCD. In Part II of this book you'll learn to remind your child that she's tougher and smarter than OCD, that OCD's victories are soon to be history. You'll team up with your child in learning all that's available about scientific advances toward recovering from this illness we call OCD. You'll help your child see his gradual improvement and express hope for deeper inroads into OCD's domain. It's not much different from the way you might learn to help a child learn to do things for herself rather than always doing things for her. Instead of colluding or fighting with the child with OCD, you become the best cheerleaders your child has ever seen. Everyone wins through this kind of teamwork.

If you end up having trouble breaking the cycle of reassuring your child about obsessions or engineering the family's day to avoid whatever triggers the obsessions, a family therapist or your child's

WHAT TO SAY TO YOUR CHILD ABOUT OCD

"How would you feel if we teamed up against OCD together? Instead of doing what OCD wants, you'll be the quarterback deciding when to resist OCD, and I'll be the cheerleader right there on the sidelines. And if we need a coach, we'll call Dr. _____."

therapist may be able to help. Support groups and associations dedicated to OCD are another important source of help for you in helping your child. These organizations serve as valuable forums for mutual acceptance, understanding, and self-discovery. They offer camaraderie with others and are clearinghouses of proven ideas for newcomers. See the Resources section at the back of the book to find support groups.

What You Need to Know about Medications for OCD

The decision to prescribe *psychotropic* medications (those that act on the brain to help the mind work properly) for children and teenagers is never made lightly. Most of them have not been studied in children as well as they have in adults, so we don't always know what positive effects and side effects they are likely to have. We may know what short-term benefits some of them have, but good long-term studies have not been done, so we don't know whether the drugs should be taken for extended periods or how even short-term use might affect a developing child's body.

This in part explains why we generally try CBT first even when OCD is severe. But if your doctor recommends medication, for any of the reasons listed in the guidelines presented earlier in the chapter, rest assured that there are several effective and reasonably safe medications to choose from. It will be up to you and the doctor to determine which one is the best medication to try first. In the following pages we sum up the latest data on these drugs—positive effects and side effects, administration and dosage, discontinuation, and combinations of medications—so that you can be an informed participant.

The medications that are generally effective and safe for OCD in children are the serotonin reuptake inhibitors (SRIs): the tricyclic antidepressant clomipramine (Anafranil), and the selective serotonin reuptake inhibitors (or SSRIs) fluoxetine (Prozac), fluvoxamine (Luvox), paroxetine (Paxil), sertraline (Zoloft), citalopram (Celexa), and escitalopram (Lexapro). What makes an SRI different from an SSRI is that the latter primarily affects serotonin, whereas the SRI clomipramine also affects other neurotransmitters, such as norepinephrine and acetylcholine. As a result, the SSRIs generally have far fewer side effects and are generally preferred. However, all of these are clearly effective for OCD in adults and apparently successful with kids, though not all have been approved by the Food and Drug Administration (FDA) for use in children.

Of these drugs, Anafranil, first released in Switzerland in 1966, was the first medication for OCD in children and adolescents. Early tests showed it to be more effective than both a placebo and desipramine, another tricyclic antidepressant. After a 1989 8-week multicenter, double-blind, parallel comparison of Anafranil and a placebo, the FDA approved it for treatment of OCD in kids and teens 10 and up. (The fact that the study was done in various locations and that neither doctors nor patients knew who was getting the active drug and who was getting a placebo—the double-blind part—made the results about as reliable as research results can be.) This study found that (1) the placebos had little or no effect; (2) improvements from the Anafranil began, on average, after 3 weeks and leveled off at 8–10 weeks; and (3) the kids and teens had an overall 37% reduction in OCD symptoms, which means "markedly to moderately" improved. Fewer than 20% of them, however, no longer had clinical OCD. These findings, which have been replicated by most other studies in children and in adults, suggest that medication is helpful but no panacea.

At the time of this writing, clomipramine is approved by the FDA for use in children with OCD, as are three of the SSRIs, which, as mentioned earlier, usually have fewer side effects than clomipramine. Here's what we know about the SSRIs to date:

- Prozac (fluoxetine): one controlled trial with children and teens clearly shows benefits for fluoxetine over placebo.
- Zoloft (sertraline): two large multicenter controlled trials, one funded by industry and one by the National Institute of Mental Health (NIMH), with children and teens show benefit for sertraline over placebo.
- Luvox (fluvoxamine): one large multicenter controlled trial with children and teens shows benefits for fluvoxamine over placebo.
- Paxil (paroxetine): Appears to be effective in children and adolescents, but perhaps with more side effects than other SSRIs. Not approved by the FDA for use in children with OCD.
- Celexa (citalopram) and Lexapro (escitalopram): Newer SSRIs are effective for OCD in adults but have not been studied systematically in children and adolescents and have not been approved for use in children or adolescents by the FDA.

Once a medication has been approved by the FDA, any doctor can legally prescribe it for any person for any reason. A responsible, competent doctor will, of course, prescribe it where it has been proven effective. But the SSRIs not yet approved by the FDA have benefited from cautious, gradual trials with children by clinicians because there was so much evidence of their effectiveness for OCD in adults. The only restriction as of this writing is that the manufacturer may not market or promote any drug for OCD in children unless it has been specifically approved for that use by the FDA.

Effectiveness

Kids, like adults, vary widely in their responses to psychotropic medications. About a third won't respond to use of a single SRI, and a second one will have to be tried. Sometimes the second medication will work when the first one didn't, but most of the time the result is the same: meaningful improvement but still symptomatic. I tell parents that these medications hit singles and doubles, not home runs, so there is no reason to cycle through multiple drug trials searching for remission. After a third SRI trial, the likelihood of getting any response at all when there has been no improvement in the first place drops considerably. It would be nice if we did, but the plain fact is that we simply don't know why a significant percentage of all children and teenagers get no benefit from these medications.

At this point you're probably wondering how to sort out all of this information. How *would* you and your doctor decide which medication to try? Because there are no direct comparisons of these medications in children or adolescents, and because the verdict in adults is that they are all equally effective on average, choices among SSRIs should be based on patient preference, personal and family medical history, and expected side effects. For example, your choice of medications may be influenced by whether someone in the family has done well or poorly with a particular medication in the past or whether the child has medical problems such as irritable stomach or sleep problems. It will also depend on the potential for drug interactions with other medications that the child may be taking. All of these factors will have to be weighed and balanced against each other to make the best first choice.

Side Effects

In general, the SSRIs are well tolerated by most people with OCD, and the side effects they do have are all similar: nervousness, insomnia, restlessness, nausea, and diarrhea. In addition, clomipramine can cause dry mouth, sedation, dizziness, and weight gain. Clomipramine is also more likely to cause problems with blood pressure and irregular heartbeats, making pretreatment and periodic electrocardiograms mandatory when using clomipramine in children and adolescents or in patients with preexisting heart disease. Occasionally, children will develop a rash, which, if it persists, will mean that the medication must be discontinued. Because the SSRIs make platelets (part of the body's blood clotting machinery) less sticky, a few children develop easy bruising or bleeding from the gums when brushing their teeth. This isn't usually a problem unless the child is playing contact sports or tends to be accident prone. A very few children will develop mania—elevated mood coupled with grandiosity, racing thoughts, decreased need for sleep, and sometimes hypersexuality—though more will become "activated" on the SSRIs. Activation is some combination of agitation, restlessness, and disinhibition, but without the grandiosity associated with mania. Mania requires that the medications be stopped and other medications for mania started; "activation" typically responds to reducing the dose of the SSRI.

Remember that all side effects are dependent on the dose of medication and on how long the child has been taking it. More severe side effects are associated with larger doses and a rapid increase in the dose. All SRIs should be withdrawn slowly because of the possibility of withdrawal reactions. The side effects also depend on body chemistry, age, other medicines your child is taking, and other medical conditions the child has. Your child's doctor will help you figure out how to manage side effects if they occur.

Although all this may sound alarming, fewer than 5% of children placed on any of the SSRIs have to discontinue the medication due to side effects. This rate compares very favorably (especially when the benefits of the medications are also considered) to other medications used in other areas of medicine, such as medicines for high blood pressure or seasonal allergies.

There has been real concern about whether the SSRIs cause children and adolescents to become suicidal or suffer particularly bad side effects when the medications are stopped. The English counterpart of the U.S. FDA (called the Medicines and Healthcare products Regulatory Agency, or MHRA) has said that doctors should not prescribe any SSRI except fluoxetine for youths with major depression. They specifically excluded children and adolescents with OCD from this restriction because these medications have been shown to be safe and effective for OCD. The U.S. FDA found that there was an increased risk of self-harm and potentially suicidal behaviors in children and adolescents treated with antidepressants, including the SSRIs. Of over 4,000 children treated in randomized controlled trials with these medications, approximately 4% became suicidal on active drug and 2% on placebo. Reassuringly, there were no completed suicides in these studies, and in our NIMH study no one became suicidal. If one were to take a single doctor treating 100 patients randomly assigned over the course of 1 year to an antidepressant and another 100 to placebo, there would be 6 clinically significant suicide-related events, 4 on active drug and 2 on placebo. Of the 4 on active medication, 2 would have happened anyway, which means that the risk difference is 2% and that about 1 in 50 would be harmed by taking the medication. Although this is far fewer than the number who

---

In another study of teenagers with depression, we found that teenagers who got CBT for depression plus fluoxetine were no more likely to experience an increase in suicidality than were teens who got CBT alone. All of the increase in suicide-related events happened in children who got medicine alone. Although this population differed from that with OCD—suicidality is much less common in OCD than in depression—findings from the Treatment for Adolescents with Depression Study (TADS), which I also led, may suggest that CBT can help protect your child from all sorts of medication-related side effects.

would benefit, it is not by any means nothing to worry about. As a result, the FDA asked antidepressant manufacturers to include in their labeling a "black box" warning statement that recommends close observation for the development of suicidality in children and adolescents treated with antidepressants for any condition, including OCD. For more up-to-date information on this topic, a very good source is *www.parentsmedguide.org*. This issue and other side effects of taking medication make it even more important that kids with OCD have the opportunity to use CBT as the sole treatment or along with medications in the treatment of OCD.

How Medications Are Administered

All of the SRIs are usually taken in pill form; fluoxetine is also available as a liquid. Except for clomipramine, which is sometimes administered twice a day or in a single bedtime dose to minimize side effects, most patients take these medications with either breakfast or dinner. The table below shows the expected dose ranges for SRIs, which vary little with age. Experts advise beginning with the equivalent of 50 mg of sertraline and waiting 2–3 weeks before increasing the dose, then moving to therapeutic doses by 6–8 weeks, for an adequate acute trial duration of 10–12 weeks. In my experience, there is little or no advantage to going to high doses, as most patients reach maximum benefit at average or below-average SRI doses if you wait long enough. Keeping the dose low and raising it slowly, with CBT on board, results in the lowest possible dose of medication and thus the minimum risk of side effects, while at the same time maximizing the chance of benefit.

Because a substantial minority of kids will not respond until 8–12 weeks have gone by, the doctor should not prescribe a new drug or add another to the treatment until at least 8 weeks have passed in which the initial medication does not seem to

SRI Dosing (in milligrams)

Drug	Usual starting	Average*	Typical range
Citalopram**	20	40	20–60
Escitalopram**	10	10	5–20
Clomipramine	50	150	200
Fluoxetine	20	40	40–60
Fluvoxamine	50	175	150–250
Paroxetine	20	30	20–40
Sertraline	50	100	150

*Average dose derived from registration trials, expert recommendation, and clinical experience.

**Not included in Expert Consensus Guidelines.

be working sufficiently. When it is apparent that a medication is not working well enough, most experts recommend switching to another SSRI. Although most patients do equally well on any of the SSRIs, some will do better on one than another, so it is important to keep trying until you find the medication that is right for your child. But again, the chances of hitting a home run decrease considerably after two failed SSRI trials, which is the time most experts recommend trying clomipramine, a tricyclic antidepressant. Sometimes adding a second medication helps boost partial response to an SRI. Your doctor can discuss this option with you, *but I believe that CBT is the most powerful augmenting treatment in part because encouragement to resist obsessions and compulsions maximizes the effectiveness of drug treatment. In this context, experts believe that complex medication strategies should be tried only when an SRI plus high-quality CBT has already been tried and failed.* Remember, changing medicine is a complicated, potentially risky decision. Don't stop your child's medicine or change the dose on your own.

WHAT TO SAY TO YOUR CHILD ABOUT OCD

"Here's how we think of your medication. It'll make OCD a bit less noisy, and that'll make it easier for you to learn the tools you need to get rid of OCD once and for all. The medication is sort of like training wheels. Once you learn how to ride a bike, you can take them off. Well, once you learn how to do the program, there's a pretty good chance you won't need to take the medication anymore."

Discuss any problems you are having with your medication with your child's doctor. Any particularly bothersome side effects or side effects that interfere with your child's normal functioning should be reported to the doctor right away.

Maintenance Treatment

When CBT or CBT plus medications proves effective, the doctor will recommend that your child switch to maintenance treatment. In maintenance treatment, the child keeps taking any medications he or she was already taking, and the visits for CBT are reduced to just enough to make sure the child keeps OCD under control. Some children who have been taking medications without CBT may have to continue taking them to prevent relapse. For example, experts recommend that anyone who has had two to four severe relapses or three or four milder relapses should be kept on long-term or even lifelong medications. The good news is that this is very uncommon when medications are combined with CBT, because CBT works better than medications and appears to offer more durable benefits when medication is stopped. When patients are doing well in maintenance, booster CBT sessions are given to prevent relapse while medications are withdrawn slowly—lowering the dose by 25%, then waiting 2 or 3 months before lowering it again, depending on the results. The idea here is to find the minimum dose of medications and of CBT that will keep symptoms at bay. For some children, this will be no medication and a yearly CBT visit. For others, some combination of low-dose SSRI and a CBT visit every 3 months will be the ticket. Whatever is necessary to keep OCD in remission is arrived at through a process of trial and error and, once set, that becomes your child's individualized treatment program.

When Nothing Works

Treatment almost always is at least a little bit helpful. Fewer than 1 in 100 children given combination treatment in our studies show no benefit. This number is 1 in 50 for those receiving CBT alone and 1 in 25 for those given medication alone. For the most part, those who don't benefit are the kids who drop out of treatment. Even those who don't go into remission are typically helped enough that they can function normally most of the time, even though OCD is still hanging around. Unfortunately, a very few children and teenagers don't seem to benefit from CBT plus an SSRI despite sticking closely with treatment. These kids, who often have multiple illnesses and complex forms of OCD, are best treated in a subspecialty OCD program that can offer treatments not typically available outside the specialty clinic setting. For example, there are CBT programs that are very intensive—50+ hours of therapist-assisted out-of-the-office CBT over 3 weeks—that take a sledgehammer to OCD. Although Marty Franklin and Edna Foa at the University of Pennsylvania have shown that the intensive program works for kids, it doesn't on average offer greater benefit than our gradual program, which we used with Drs. Foa and Franklin in our research study. But for the really sick child who hasn't benefited from weekly CBT plus medications, it can be a lifesaver. A very few children (I've seen only 2 in 15 years) need hospitalization for OCD, so if your doctor recommends hospitalization, it will probably be for some other reason. Most kids don't need heroic treatments, but we mention them only so that you know what your options are if more standard routes don't work for your child.

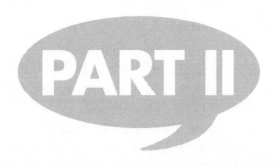

Eight Steps for Getting Rid of Obsessions and Compulsions

IF YOU'RE A KID WITH OCD, this part of the book is for you. In the next eight chapters are proven steps for running OCD out of your life. You may end up working through these steps with your therapist, but you might also be able to handle them on your own, with help from your parents. How much help you're going to need is something you, your parents, and your doctor should talk about before you begin. You want to give yourself the best possible chance of succeeding with this program right from the start.

First, though, read through Chapters 5–12 (read the first section of each chapter, which is just for you, and the parents' sections that follow if you want). If you have any questions about the program as you read, stop and talk to your parents (and your therapist if you're seeing one regularly). When you've finished, your parents should sit down with you and talk about whether to do the program and how you think it should go. Maybe you'll feel your strongest if you have a therapist work with you at first, then go it alone once you feel comfortable starting to talk back to OCD.

The whole program will take somewhere between 3 and 5 months. If that sounds like a long time to you, think about what a pain it's been to get through every day with OCD around. If you can make OCD stop bothering you, 3 to 5 months of "homework" is nothing, and it may be less if OCD is mild and you get the hang of it quickly.

Here's a quick look at what you'll be doing (based on 3 months—but you may add a week or two to each segment if you need it):

• *Weeks 1 and 2*: You'll really get the idea that OCD is a medical illness—a brain hiccup—not some sort of craziness or badness in you. You'll learn to tell the difference between the stuff in your head that comes from OCD and the thoughts and feelings that come from the good, smart kid that you are. By the end of the second week or so, you'll be an expert at spotting OCD's tricks. Most important, you'll have a road map to OCD that tells you how and where you can start doing the opposite of what OCD says.

• *Weeks 3-10*: You'll learn to resist, or talk back to, OCD whenever it tries to pull its usual tricks on you. You'll take it nice and slow so you'll know you're safe but fast enough to show OCD you mean business and won't be playing its games anymore. It'll be kind of like learning to watch scary TV shows. One girl I know wanted to watch all the horror movies on TV around Halloween like the other kids but was really afraid of them. So she started out turning them on but only listening to them from another room. Then she'd sit on the couch in front of the TV—but with a blanket over her head. Then she started pulling the blanket away from one eye. Finally she watched a movie with both eyes. To this day she still has a blanket on her lap just in case things get too scary, but she watches the whole movie. While you're learning them, the skills taught in this program are going to be like that blanket for you. You'll have them available anytime OCD tries to bug you again so you can keep talking back to OCD without getting too scared or uncomfortable to stick it out. Then you'll drop the blanket altogether because you'll have learned to make that brain hiccup that is OCD turn itself off.

• *Weeks 11-12*: Here's where you learn to make sure you're protected if OCD ever tries to come back. You'll learn to recognize the warning signs that OCD is trying to get back into your life and what you can do instantly to seal up that crack in your armor. We'll give you a practice schedule for keeping up your defenses—kind of like exercising to make sure you don't lose your muscles after being in training for a sport.

Once you're ready to get started, this is what you'll do:

1. Read through the chapter. Talk to your parents and/or therapist about what is required, and be sure to mention anything that's not clear to you.
2. Follow the instructions for learning the skills.
3. Do the homework! You won't get anywhere unless you stay on top of homework assignments.
4. Make sure you're ready to move on before you go to the next step.

While you're doing all this, *ask for help* if you ever feel stuck. After your section of each chapter is a section for your parents so they'll know what they can do to help you and how they can avoid accidentally making things harder (you know they mean well, but they started out just as clueless about OCD as you did). Some kids just back off when they feel bullied by OCD, and this only encourages OCD. We're going to give you ideas to make sure you ask for help in getting unstuck instead. In case you ever have trouble admitting you're feeling overwhelmed, in the parent sections we'll clue Mom and Dad in to the signs that you're having trouble so they can offer help if you ever find it impossible to ask for it.

But here's the most important thing to remember about the way this program works: *You're in charge.* It's about time, isn't it? For a while now, OCD has been kind of ruling your life. And your parents probably haven't been able to help you get rid of OCD. That's because the only person who can talk back to OCD is you. You've been the one OCD has been bossing around, and it's up to you to do the bossing back. So the whole program is about giving you the power to do that. You can get all the help you need. But you're the one who learns and uses the skills. You're the one who sets the pace. You're the one who chalks up the wins against OCD.

Ready to get going on that?

A brief word about doing the homework: We know more homework probably feels like the last thing you need or want. But just like the homework you get at school, if you don't do the homework here, you won't really get good at what you've been taught. Most kids do the homework assigned at school so they'll get a good report card and make their parents happy and feel like they're achieving something to be proud of. Here you have a lot to gain by doing the homework: getting rid of OCD.

If you practice the skills taught in each step, you'll get closer and closer to running OCD out of your life. If you don't practice them, OCD will stay in charge. But don't worry about your "grades." All you need to do is make steady progress. Sometimes you'll move slowly, sometimes fast, and most of the time in the middle. Some tasks you'll be assigned will be so quick and easy to do that you may not think of it as home*work* at all. Others will require some stick-to-itiveness, but this book and your parents, along with your therapist if you have one, will help you get there.

Also, the program provides graphs and charts to use because many kids find them helpful. They help you keep track of that steady progress you're making so you know the effort is worthwhile. But if you're one of those kids who find writing a chore, this is a good place to call in Mom or Dad to help. Your parents can be your recordkeeper (kind of like the way many parents volunteer to keep the stats at your basketball or soccer game) if you're comfortable with that (remember, you're in charge here). If not, and you don't think the writing we suggest in various steps is going to help you, just skip it.

The OCD Toolkit

Tools You'll Use to Talk Back to OCD

• A nickname for OCD: Using this name (or just the illness's name) for OCD from now on will remind you that OCD *is not you* and can be run out of your life. (Chapter 5)

• Your symptom/hiccup chart (map): This is a chart where you fill in your symptoms so you can talk back to OCD in each place it bugs you until it goes away one place at a time. You'll keep updating this from Step 2 and all the way through. (Chapter 6)

• Fear thermometer: This is a tool for measuring how uncomfortable OCD makes you feel when you have to deal with a specific "hiccup" on your symptom chart (above). It will help you figure out which symptoms to resist OCD in first and will be used to help you know how long to resist OCD every time you do the "talking back" practice that is the main work of the program. (Chapter 6)

• Small spiral notebook for taking notes about your experiences in talking back to OCD so you know what to do the same or differently in the next step. (Chapter 7)

• Brainpower techniques: Ways to change the way you think about OCD that help you remember that it's all nonsense and doesn't need to be taken seriously. (Chapter 7)

- Scouting OCD to see where you can "win" easily.
- Giving yourself a pep talk: Be kind to yourself and don't get down on yourself when OCD is hard to boss back.
- Cutting OCD down to size: Examine OCD's claims to show yourself how silly they are.
- Letting OCD float by: Remember that OCD is just something out there that passes through and then is gone, like a thunderstorm—we'll teach you how to just let it go by.

• Brainpower card: A list of the brainpower techniques that shows which ones work best for you and that may also list some "lines" you can deliver in the script that makes *you* the author of your encounters with OCD. Carry this card with you, and you can pull it out as a reminder of what to do when OCD takes you by surprise and you want to remember how to talk back. (Chapter 7)

• Rewards: You and your parents agree on rewards that you earn for progress made against OCD. Everybody needs rewards for hard work to keep them going. (Chapter 7)

• The work zone: Your list of symptoms that have fear temperature of 2-3, meaning that you can talk back to OCD successfully at least half of the time. These are the symptoms that become your tasks to tackle when you start seriously talking back to OCD. (Chapter 8)

• EX/RP: Exposure and response prevention, the most important tool of all, the key to talking back to OCD in earnest. It's a way to face a hiccup and wait OCD out without doing the usual ritual. With practice, it shows OCD that you're not falling for its tricks anymore and helps you get rid of OCD symptoms one by one. (Chapter 8)

• EX/RP task lists: "Ladders" that break one tough symptom down into increasingly harder tasks that you can tackle one at a time until the symptom is gone. (Chapter 8)

• Task records: A form you can use, if you want, to keep track of your lowering fear temperature during an EX/RP task. If you don't like to write, don't bother with this form. (Chapter 8)

• Four ways to break OCD's rules: These are ways to talk back even when OCD is making it tough. (Chapter 9)

- Delay the ritual.
- Shorten the ritual.
- Do the ritual differently.
- Do the ritual slowly.

• Chill-out skills: Ways to hang in there in an EX/RP task when you feel uncomfortable enough that you're tempted to bail out. (Chapter 9)

- Deep breathing
- Relaxation

• Notifications and ceremonies: Announcements and celebrations (in addition to the more frequent rewards) that acknowledge major leaps forward in talking back to OCD so you realize how far you've come. (Chapter 10)

• 10 guidelines for keeping OCD out of your life: You can write these down on a card to carry with you when you've finished the program, to remind you of what you've achieved and how to maintain your gains. (Chapter 12)

Tools You'll Use to Keep Track of Your Progress through the Program

• The Taking Stock Scale: This is a way to measure how much trouble OCD is causing you. You'll use it at the end of each step to help you see how much headway you're making against OCD.

• The Taking Stock Graph: Here you plot the numbers from the Taking Stock

Scale at the end of each step, making a line graph that will show you how your strength is rising while OCD's is falling.

• "Getting Stronger Every Day" forms: These are just a way to keep track of the fact that you're doing your *Talking Back to OCD* homework every day. Seeing that they're sticking with the program helps some kids keep going. But if you don't like this kind of paperwork, you don't have to use these forms—or you can let your parents keep these records if you want. They appear at the end of the kids' section of Chapter 5, 9, 10, and 12.

• Summary sheets for each step: These are just lists of the tasks you'll do during each step, which you can post where you'll see them as a reminder to keep talking back to OCD. If you don't think they'll help you, don't use them. They're in an appendix at the back of the book.

5

Step 1: What Kind of Treatment Is This, Anyway?

THE PROGRAM YOU'RE ABOUT TO BEGIN is built on years of research by doctors who specialize in the treatment of kids with OCD. It is the only proven therapy for OCD, and it works really well, even better than medications. First developed in research clinics, it has been used by many therapists and kids just like you to help children and teenagers toss OCD out of their lives. Now it's *your* program too. This chapter will tell you how to use it.

Each chapter in the program is divided into these sections:

- "The Game Plan": This summary tells you what you'll be doing during the step covered in the chapter. It also gives you some tips for success and helps you review what you did in the last step so you're reminded of what you've accomplished and so you're sure you're ready to go forward. Read the game plan first to be sure you're prepared for the step.
- "Get Ready": This section tells you what you need to do before launching into the real tasks of the step.
- "Get Going": Here's where you'll find the instructions for the step.
- "Taking Stock": At the end of the step you'll see how you're doing, using some tools that will show you in pictures how quickly you're progressing.

You may think you know a lot of what you'll read already, and many kids actually do know much more about OCD than their doctors do. But try to do each step with a "beginner's mind." Doing all of the program will give you the best chance of mastering the tools you need to get rid of OCD.

The Game Plan for Step 1

1. *The first thing you're going to work on is to stop being so hard on yourself.* Being kind to yourself about OCD is incredibly important. I know you've been trying to get rid of OCD in your own way for quite a while now. The fact that it hasn't worked is not your fault. You just didn't have the right tools. You'll get them in this program. For now, take a deep breath and tell yourself you're not to blame for OCD. This chapter will show you how to believe that.

2. *Do the reading and other preparation listed under "Get Ready."*

3. *Follow the instructions for Step 1, planning to spend about a week on this step.* You'll be adding in Step 2 this week and Steps 3 and 4 next week. In fact, for the first four steps, which overlap, 2 weeks is more than enough in most cases. Quicker is OK if you've really got it, and a little slower is OK if you need the extra time. Work with your parents and/or your therapist as needed. Post the "Getting Stronger Every Day" chart (shown at the end of this chapter) for Steps 1-4 where you'll see it easily and check off the fact that you've done the homework at the end of each day. Exactly when you add Steps 2-4 is up to you, as long as you aim for doing all four steps during the first 2 weeks of the program. The point of checking off when you add each step is just to help you remember to do so, not to "grade" you on how quickly you move forward.

4. *After 4 days or so, take stock.* Be sure you feel comfortable before going on to Step 2 (or 3 if you've added Step 2 during this first week).

Get Ready

If you haven't done so already, read Part I of this book or ask your parents to go over it with you. Everything you'll learn there about the illness called OCD lays an important foundation for the work you're about to begin. Think of it as an important part of retraining your brain not to hiccup anymore. Post the summary sheet for this step (at the back of the book) where you can see it easily—inside your bedroom door or somewhere else you'll pass by often.

Get Going

Gather Your Team or Allies: New Roles for a New Game Plan

All you do in this first task is get used to the idea that you and the people who want to help you get rid of OCD are going to play new roles. If there is one thought we want you to hold on to while going through this program, it's that *you are in charge.* You will be calling the shots—deciding which parts of OCD to go after when and setting the pace for progress. If you've done your reading of Part I, you know we want you to think of your family and friends and your doctor, if you have one, as a team working together against this illness we call OCD. Let's say you're involved in a competition against OCD, one that our program will train you to win. Every player will have an important role, and the team's chances of winning will increase when everyone does his or her job. As Mike Krzyzewski, Duke University's exceptionally successful basketball coach, says, a team is like a fist. Each finger plays an important role, but it's the whole that's the key to success. The key point that Mike makes is that this is our team, with everyone playing his or her part.

You: The Young Person with OCD

Think of yourself as the point guard, the captain, the quarterback, the admiral, the pilot, or whatever title appeals to you. The point is you're in charge. Gradually you'll take control over OCD; for now, though, try to think of yourself as learning how to be in control of the game or battle plan for fighting OCD. You won't get there all at once, but over the next few weeks you'll get comfortable in this role as you learn what to do to talk back to OCD. To start, know that you're not the problem—OCD is—and also that you're not bad, crazy, or alone. You're a normal person who just happens to have this particular illness we call OCD.

As the boss, you'll be equipped with lots of tools and skills that you and your family will find very useful in turning the tables on OCD. We'll describe that "toolkit" later in this chapter. For now, what's important to know is that one of your new tools will put you in charge by helping you judge the difficulty of resisting OCD so that you make progress without trying to go too far too fast. This isn't a "just say no" program—you would have done that already if you could, so don't worry about having to do the impossible. You'll get there, but only as fast as what works for you. Parents, other family members, and maybe a therapist will be available to help you keep going, but they won't push you to do something you simply cannot do.

> *Every time I was able to resist OCD, my dad wanted me to quit it altogether. But when we learned that OCD is like going up a ladder one step at a time, Dad and I were back on the same team again.*
>
> *—John, age 10*

Other tools will teach you how to become your own biggest fan—and help you stay that way even when the going gets tough. If you're like most kids, you've probably been down on yourself for being unable to stop doing OCD. When you've tried to resist OCD's demands, thoughts like "I won't be able to do this" and "I'm such a disaster" probably popped into your head, and they may have convinced you to perform even more time-consuming rituals to fight your fears than before. This, of course, only made you feel worse about yourself. Now we're going to help you learn to say, instead, "Resisting OCD will be tough, but using my toolkit, I can do it right here, right now." As we're about to explain, "right here, right now" soon becomes "again," and before long facing down any particular OCD symptom is as easy as tying your shoes. By the way, that's true even if OCD has you and your shoes tied up in knots.

Another way that you'll stay in charge is by learning to use your brainpower to its fullest. This means becoming an expert—on OCD in general and on your version of OCD in particular. If you had asthma, your family would help you understand how to take care of yourself so you could continue to play sports, dance, swim, and pursue all the other activities that asthma can make difficult. You'd learn about what causes asthma, what triggers an attack, and what kind of preventive measures and treatments will help. You'd also learn about all the signs and signals of an asthma attack that are unique to you and how to ask for help when you need it.

This is what we'll be asking of you regarding OCD: Educate yourself, with your parents' help as needed, about OCD and all the strides we keep making toward curing it. Also, to beat OCD at its own game, you have to get to know OCD as it affects you in great detail. We call this "mapping OCD," and it means becoming aware of exactly how, when, and where OCD interferes in your life so you can head it off and defeat it when it shows up. You especially have to learn how to recognize where you win sometimes and where OCD wins sometimes. Your map will show you that so you can decide when and where to fight back—how to turn winning some-times into winning all the time. This map will also help your parents know when to help and when to back off with respect to resisting OCD. Your map of OCD is an important tool that we'll talk a little more about later in the chapter.

Your Parents

It's pretty simple: Your parents may be in charge of other aspects of your life because you're still a kid (even if you're a teenager), but in this game they'll have to learn to follow your lead. Your parents will be your greatest cheerleaders, but they won't serve as coach or manager. That's the job of this program, which they've signed on to. They can offer support and help, especially when you ask for it. They'll get you a therapist if you need one and don't have one. They'll help you keep moving forward with the program, without doing any of the work for you. They're going to cheer you on and start paying more attention to all the things that are going great than to OCD.

Other Family Members

Your brothers and sisters could become part of your team too, especially if they're tangled up in OCD along with you. But even if they're not participating in rituals or getting involved with OCD in some other way, they can be pretty good cheerleaders, like your parents. Mom or Dad or your therapist should be in charge of helping them know what their new role will be.

Therapists, Doctors, and Other Helpers

If you already have a therapist, you and your parents will want to mention that you'd like to try this program and see how the therapist might want to be involved. Your therapist should be available to jump in and help you get unstuck as needed. We'll point to the signs that you need a little assistance in sections called "How a Therapist Can Help." But anytime you feel stuck and need more than your parents' support, you should call your therapist or have your parents call.

Your Teachers

Whether your teachers end up being part of the team depends on how OCD is affecting your life at school. If your teachers already know you have OCD and have been helpful to you, consider them part of the team. Talk to your parents about meeting with the teachers to let them in on the game plan.

Support Groups

There are lots of other kids out there with OCD, and sometimes sharing your struggles can make you all feel better. Other kids and their parents can also give you ideas you may not have thought of for getting around OCD when things get sticky. If you think you'd like to meet some of these other kids, check the Resources at the back of this book.

Get a Picture of the Whole Program

Your job here is simply to familiarize yourself with what you're going to be doing in the eight steps. Either you've read about the type of treatment used in this program in Chapter 4 or your parents have explained it to you. Remember, the basic idea is that you make your brain stop hiccupping OCD by changing what you do in relation to what OCD seems to demand of you. Instead of doing what OCD wants (like washing your hands over and over or steering clear of anything that seems germy), you face the germs or other scary thing *on purpose*. And when you do, you don't do whatever usually makes you feel better, like washing your hands. You don't change all at once, everywhere OCD is involved with your life. We'll show you how to do it slowly but surely, at your own pace, so you don't get so freaked out that you want to back off completely.

Hard to believe this will work? Doing it will show you it works. But most kids naturally don't feel like taking this risk. After all, they've tried to resist OCD before, without much luck. So another part of the program teaches the whole family a new way of thinking and talking about OCD. This new way of thinking about OCD gives you all confidence that you can call the shots and take control of your lives back from OCD.

Changing what you do and what you think in this way can help people do all kinds of things that may seem impossible, from losing weight to quitting smoking to getting over a fear of spiders. And it can help you resist OCD. The "secret weapon" is the "toolkit" we mentioned earlier, which makes both acting differently and thinking differently work even better.

Your toolkit will spell out ways to handle the fear and other uncomfortable feelings OCD brings on. The toolkit includes your "map" of OCD—a picture of the parts of your life where OCD doesn't interfere at all, where it interferes a lot, and where it's there but not all the time because you can control your response to it. This territory, where OCD is around but hasn't taken over completely, where you already resist successfully some of the time, is what we call the *work zone*. It is a lot easier to change winning some of the time to winning all of the time than it is to go from winning none of the time to all of the time. That's why it's in the parts of your life where you're already winning that you're going to work on resisting OCD. After all, you already have some power here, so you stand a 100% chance of triumphing over OCD—with the help of your toolkit.

Another important tool is something we call the *fear thermometer*. You use this to make sure nothing you try to resist is either so hard that you won't succeed or so easy that it won't really convince OCD you're serious about running it out of town. With these two tools, plus lots of other skills that go in the kit, you can stick with the program and be finished in just a few months.

As you read in Chapter 1, OCD is like a broken switch in your brain, which makes it hard to stop worrying even when there's really nothing to fear. By changing the way you respond to OCD and using your toolkit, you learn to turn off the OCD hiccup in your brain by standing your ground for just a little while longer than usual, even though OCD wants you to run away or do a ritual like washing your hands 10 times. You stick out the fear for a little longer each day, and eventually your brain gets so used to it that you don't even notice anymore. Switch fixed! OCD gone.

You've probably already had this kind of thing happen to you many times before. I knew one young man who rented an apartment right next to the elevated train tracks in Chicago and found the noise of the passing trains deafening for a couple of weeks. Because he had no place else to live, he couldn't just move out, so he stayed. Within weeks, he told me, he no longer noticed the noise at all. Friends would come to visit and say "How can you stand that noise?" when the first train went by, and the young man found himself replying "What noise?" His brain turned the noise off. Right now your brain has OCD on full volume. You can turn OCD off by facing it directly and gradually doing the opposite of what it tells you. We know it sounds silly—you've been trying to resist OCD ever since it first popped up—but within a very few months, if you follow this program, chances are you won't even hear OCD anymore.

I knew a girl named Angela who didn't believe she'd ever be able to resist OCD. Just resisting a little bit sounded like it would be far too scary to her. But she was also on her junior high swim team, where she was pretty good at the high dives. I told her to think about how she got to the point where she could dive off that high board: First she swam in the shallow end, then the deep end. Then she jumped off the side of the pool, then the low board. Then, first really nervously and then without even thinking about it, she jumped off the high dive. Finally she learned to go headfirst. That's how this program works—one step at a time. Knowing that helped Angela stop assuming she'd be too scared to do this program and start the first step.

How a therapist can help: If you have lots of questions about how this type of program works or feel really worried about how it will go for you, your therapist is the best person to answer your questions. It's important to feel confident that you can do this before you start. You know how it is: When you're really worried that you don't know the math that's going to be on the quiz, you're pretty likely not to do so well—even if you really do know the stuff backward and forward. Talk to your therapist so you'll feel better about what you're about to do.

Give OCD a Funny Nickname or Learn to Call It by Its Medical Name

For this task, which is the foundation of everything that follows, you start refer-
ring to OCD as something that's not part of you. The truth is, *OCD is not you.* OCD worms its way into the brain as if it belongs there, so it's no wonder that many kids have trouble figuring out where OCD ends and they begin. It has nothing to do with

you, though, any more than hiccups do. OCD is your brain on hiccups, and your job is to deal with it, not blame yourself for it. We'll say it again: OCD is not you, has no meaning, isn't personal. It is just a brain hiccup that unfortunately you've got to deal with.

One way to remember that OCD is just something that happens, like the hiccups or the weather, is to give OCD a funny nickname. Or, if you're to old for something like this, just call OCD by its medical name. By naming it for what it is you make it separate from you. Having made it "not you," you can hold it out away from yourself, see it clearly for what it is—just a hiccup that has no particular meaning or value—and deal with it skillfully so it goes away and stops bothering you. Ditto for your parents, teachers, anyone who has been blaming you for what looks like crazy bad behavior but is really just the illness we call OCD.

Can you come up with a name for OCD that shows it for what it is—annoying but surprisingly weak once you know how to deal with it? Let's cut OCD down to size. Once you choose a nickname, you and your parents should use that name whenever you're talking about obsessions and compulsions: "Old Pain in the Butt is at it again." "Mr. Stinky keeps trying to make me listen to him today." "Dirtball won't let me anywhere near the garbage cans today."

If using a name like this seems silly, just start calling OCD *OCD*, the way you call the flu *the flu*. It's not personal; it's medical. "OCD won't let me finish washing my hands today." "OCD keeps trying to tell me what to do!" Whether you call it OCD or by another name, practice talking about OCD as though it's a third person in the room until you get really used to doing that.

Instead of:	Say:
"I have to line up my shoes before I can go to school."	"Neat Freak is trying to get me to hang around this closet all morning."
"Are you sure that glass is clean?"	"OCD is telling me there are lots of germs in that glass."
"I'm always thinking bad things."	"Mr. Nag is scolding me again—but those ideas are his, not mine!"
"If I don't count everything in the right order, I'll have to start all over."	"Math Nerd is such a pain."
"I can't touch anything in the library without gloves."	"OCD makes me feel really scared of touching things that might have other people's germs."

Start Noticing Where OCD Wins and Where You Win

For the next week, try to notice those places where you win sometimes and OCD wins sometimes. By the time they start this program, many families feel that OCD rules their lives. They stop noticing that OCD in fact is not in control all or even most of the time. An awful lot of life actually goes on without OCD at all, though it may seem like OCD invades everything. If you pay attention, you'll realize there are plenty of times when you win against OCD: An obsession comes up, and for whatever reason, you're able to shove aside the thought, or just let OCD come and go and ignore OCD's demands. This is where we fight back—where you win sometimes and lose sometimes. Anything easier wouldn't be worth it; anything harder is impossible, at least for now. Hard things become easier as you go through the program. To understand this, you have to pay attention to how OCD works.

So, for the next week or so, try to notice when and where you win sometimes and OCD wins sometimes. Compare those situations to the times and places where OCD wins most or all of the time. Also try to notice what else is going on at the time. What makes it easier to resist OCD? What makes it harder? Are you happy at the time when OCD is winning? Or are you mad? Does it matter? How easy is it not to get lost in OCD—that is, to keep it named as something different from you that you can simply look at without getting involved? Don't think about who has the "higher score" at this point. Pretend you're a reporter or a private eye. Simply watch what happens and when it happens. In doing this exercise, always use the name you chose for OCD. Besides helping you keep your distance from OCD, that will help you avoid worrying about whether you're doing the program "right." Right now you want to learn something about how OCD works, but you also just want to get good at seeing what's happening between you and OCD without blaming. You can even watch how wanting to get rid of OCD makes you frustrated and how this can make OCD harder to resist. Why? Because getting frustrated and upset strengthens OCD. Learning not to take OCD personally—just as you wouldn't take asthma or arthritis personally—makes the program much easier to follow. Besides, there's no one to blame (except OCD) anyway.

Taking Stock

OK, you've followed the instructions for taking some new and important steps against OCD. How did it go? Do you find yourself thinking a little differently about OCD? Instead of getting upset about how bad you feel, do you find yourself saying "Well, here come those hiccups again" or "Germy was such a pain today"? If someone asked what you were going to do over the next few days, would you have a pretty good idea of what the plan is and where you're headed with this program? Have you started to realize that OCD isn't in charge of your *whole* life after all?

If you can say yes to a couple of these—or even "maybe"—you're on the right track and ready to keep going. You'll keep doing what you've done in this step while you add Step 2, the next chapter. In the meantime, record where you stand with OCD on the following form and then start making a graph on the page that follows. You're going to add to it after each step.

Here's a great way to see how you're doing at the end of each step. Circle the number that matches what's going on with you and OCD now that you're at the end of the step. The higher the number, the more of a pain OCD is for you. Next, plot the number on the following graph.

1
2 OCD is hardly around at all. I don't have to spend much time resisting it, and it doesn't get in the way of whatever I want and need to do during the day.
3

4 OCD is there, and we all know it. But I spend only a little time on OCD every day. OCD is
5 easy to resist and doesn't really cause my family or anyone else a big problem.
6

7 I spend a pretty big part of my day dealing with OCD. It's hard not to think about OCD
8 and what it wants me to do. Mom, Dad, and others have to help me stay on track with
9 school, chores, and even fun stuff; otherwise I miss out on some things because of OCD.

10 OCD pretty much rules my day. If Mom and Dad and other people didn't help me, I
11 wouldn't get anything else done, except obeying OCD's commands. It often feels like I
12 spend my whole day on rituals.

13 I can't do anything on my own. OCD makes it hard for me to eat dinner like everyone
14 else, get dressed, go where I want to go in my house, and even sleep all night. I feel like I
15 can't make a move without OCD bossing me around, and Mom, Dad, and my doctors
     have to help me do almost everything.

Taking Stock: Graphing Your Progress

Plot the number you chose for your experience with OCD following each step. Keep the graph handy so you can see how far you've come once you've completed the first few steps.

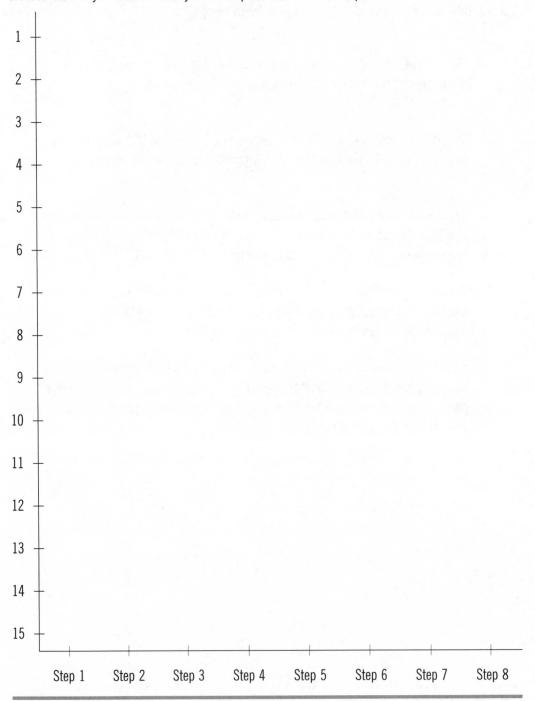

At the end of each day, check off whether you've followed the instructions for the step. Also check off the point when you started adding Steps, 2, 3, and 4, just to remind yourself to add in these steps during the first 2 weeks. (We divided up the 2 weeks pretty evenly, but you may end up adding the next step a little sooner or a little later; just keep track so you know where you are in the program.)

Day 1 ☐ I did the homework for Step 1.

Day 2 ☐ I did the homework for Step 1.

Day 3 ☐ I did the homework for Step 1.

Day 4 ☐ I did the homework for Step 1.
☐ I did the homework for Step 2.

Day 5 ☐ I did the homework for Step 1.
☐ I did the homework for Step 2.

Day 6 ☐ I did the homework for Step 1.
☐ I did the homework for Step 2.

Day 7 ☐ I did the homework for Step 1.
☐ I did the homework for Step 2.

Day 8 ☐ I did the homework for Step 1.   ☐ I did the homework for Step 3.
☐ I did the homework for Step 2.

Day 9 ☐ I did the homework for Step 1.   ☐ I did the homework for Step 3.
☐ I did the homework for Step 2.

Day 10 ☐ I did the homework for Step 1.   ☐ I did the homework for Step 3.
☐ I did the homework for Step 2.

Day 11 ☐ I did the homework for Step 1.   ☐ I did the homework for Step 3.
☐ I did the homework for Step 2.   ☐ I did the homework for Step 4.

Day 12 ☐ I did the homework for Step 1.   ☐ I did the homework for Step 3.
☐ I did the homework for Step 2.   ☐ I did the homework for Step 4.

Day 13 ☐ I did the homework for Step 1.   ☐ I did the homework for Step 3.
☐ I did the homework for Step 2.   ☐ I did the homework for Step 4.

Day 14 ☐ I did the homework for Step 1.   ☐ I did the homework for Step 3.
☐ I did the homework for Step 2.   ☐ I did the homework for Step 4.

Step 1: Instructions for Parents

READ THE FOLLOWING SECTION in full before your child starts on Step 1. You may not need all of this information, but much of it will come in handy when you need to give your child a little morale boost. Everything in this section parallels the kids' section for the step. In many cases it's helpful for kids to read the parent instructions too, by the way, so your child knows without a doubt that you'll be putting the reins in his hands while being there to support and encourage every step of the way.

If your son or daughter who has OCD is a teenager, feel your way carefully and ask—don't tell—whether he or she needs any help in getting started. Teenagers should be able to jump right in and take control, but you know your child best, and some teens will need some encouragement to get started.

With younger kids, it's best to gently monitor their reading of the chapter up to "Get Going." Have them stop at that point and tell you what they think; ask if they have any questions. When they seem ready (they should seem at least willing, if not raring to go), have them start with the first task. Here, too, feel your way. If you get the idea that your child will have a hard time being a self-starter, offer to talk through the goal and the homework with him or her. Just be very careful not to do the work yourself. Always let your child take the lead, keep reminding the child that he or she is in charge, and congratulate your son or daughter for taking any step toward that goal.

If your child needs it, offer gentle reminders to keep working through the chapter. For example, make it a habit to check your child's "Getting Stronger Every Day" chart and say "I bet it feels great to see what you've accomplished!" every time you notice that the child has checked off having done the homework for the day. If you start noticing forward progress in this way, you'll then be able to ask gently "Did you forget to check off today on your chart?" when you see this hasn't been done. Assuming that your child just forgot to do the record keeping opens the door for your child to tell you whether the homework in fact was done—and if not, where he or she may be having trouble that you can help with.

Solid progress should be made during the first week, and many kids will be ready to start Step 2 during the same week. Once your child completes a task (such as giving OCD a nickname), move on to the next, making sure that everyone in the family is integrating the accomplished goal into daily life. Don't be overzealous about this, though. You want to demonstrate that doing these tasks will make life easier for the child with OCD and for everyone else, not put more pressure on the family. So if family members get a slow start in changing how they refer to OCD, don't nag or correct them but rather simply model the right way to talk about it:

TYLER: Mom, Dylan's using up all the towels in the bathroom again!
MOM: Boy, old Fussbudget sure makes a lot of laundry for us, doesn't he?

MOM: Dylan, you're going to make us all late for the movie!
DAD: Hey, Dylan, is Fussbudget giving you a really hard time right now?

At the end of the week, participate in taking stock with your child, or ask your teenager how it went. This will give you a chance to make sure the pace is appropriate and also to offer your praise and encouragement for a job well done.

The Game Plan for Step 1

1. The first task for everyone in the family before starting this program is to wipe the slate clean. Typically, neither children who have been struggling with OCD nor their families feel particularly powerful or effective at this point. All that is about to change. We're going to supply what your child needs to succeed against OCD, but these tools won't be as effective as they can be if undercurrents of guilt and frustration flow through all your interactions. You just won't be able to help your child if you're distracted in that way, so get ready to wipe the slate clean, which you'll learn to do here with an open mind, just as your son or daughter is learning to do.

2. Wiping the slate clean means turning control of how you respond to OCD over to this program. Make sure you and your child do the reading and other preparation listed under "Get Ready."

3. Your child should feel pretty comfortable with each step before going to the next one, and depending on his or her age, you may have to monitor progress closely to ensure that the timing is right. For the first four steps, 2 weeks is more than enough in most cases. Taking more than 3 weeks for Steps 1–4 generally means that the child needs a therapist's help, at least at first. Don't nag, but do observe closely.

Hannah has pretty severe germ worries and washing rituals. She started the program on her own, with the help of her parents. However, despite a really firm commitment to make the program work (as outlined in our book for therapists), by week 3 she was stuck and feeling discouraged. Her parents were frustrated (as was Hannah) because they'd started the work with high hopes. Doing the skillful thing, no one blamed anybody. Instead, they sought out a cognitive-behavioral therapist who was experienced with OCD. He saw immediately that Hannah had not really mastered the art of talking to herself about OCD correctly and that this was due to a kind of OCD that involved "doubting." With a correction that involved naming doubting as OCD, Hannah got back on track and within 4 months was mostly free of OCD symptoms.

4. After 1 week, make sure your child takes stock as described. Again, each goal should take about a week to introduce and practice before moving to the next goal. However, for a variety of reasons, this sometimes doesn't happen—it may go quickly or more slowly—so the basic principle is that kids should be sure they feel comfortable before going on to the next step.

A caution: Don't assume that immediate success means that you should push ahead faster. Let your child dictate the pace of progress, especially early on. Failure that comes from trying to go too far too soon tends to breed discouragement and frustration.

Get Ready

Your son or daughter needs to acquire the background knowledge provided by Part I as much as you do. The trick will be for you to assess the child's ability to read and assimilate this information on his or her own. If your child is 10–12 (the age the kids' instructions are generally aimed at) or older and a reasonably good reader, he or she could very well read this independently. If younger, you'll have to take the lead. Read the section yourself. Then go back and look at the "What to Say to Your Child about OCD . . ." boxes for some ideas for explaining the concepts to your child. Your child's reactions will give you a good idea of his or her readiness to work through this program and the level of help likely to be needed. Be sure to read the quotes from other kids to your child if he or she isn't reading Part I independently; they really give kids a sense of solidarity with others going through the same struggles.

Get Going

Gather Your Team or Allies: New Roles for a New Game Plan

If everyone is to stop behaving like OCD's puppets, the way things are done at home needs to change first. This means a shift in roles for everyone.

Your family is going to be working together against OCD. Some families I've worked with like to think of themselves as armies waging a battle against OCD. Others prefer something gentler, like being on a sports team or simply working together to cure an illness. I like the *Karate Kid* movies, where the young man learns wisdom skills that involve calmly using the opponent's weaknesses to defeat him, but what is appropriate for your child will be up to you and your child.

As you read in the Introduction to this book, your role will be quite different from what you've been doing up to this point and may even seem to go against the grain of parental authority and protection. You may be used to taking the reins, but instead we are going to ask you to step back and go with the program outlined in this book. You'll be asked to stop some things you're now doing and to start doing some things you're not doing. In each case, your role will be to help your child solve a problem that can be solved only when the child, rather than her parents, plays the central role in resisting OCD. Each step on the path to triumphing over OCD will give you specific suggestions regarding how to help skillfully, but it all boils down to the following changes in attitude and behavior toward the child with OCD:

- *Work on always speaking about OCD using the nickname your child chose.* It may feel awkward, and it will take practice, but by referring to OCD as a third person in the room, or even better, as something impersonal, such as the weather, you'll help yourself and your child see OCD as it is: a meaningless brain hiccup separate from your child, not something that has to be taken at face value. Modeling this new way of talking about OCD will help your child understand that OCD is not the same as her as a person.

- *Practice kindness, generosity, and patience.* Always treat your child as you would if he or she had a medical illness such as asthma or arthritis. Remember, no one hates OCD more than your child does. OCD is a plague on your planet, but your child can begin resisting OCD only at the point at which she is already sometimes successful in beating OCD. This book will go to great lengths to help you find that spot, so you know exactly what is over and done with, where to resist rituals, and where to practice patience and kindness. We tend to think of patience as "grin and bear it" endurance, but really it's the willingness and ability to accept with kindness what can't for the moment be fixed. When you're frustrated that OCD is still hanging around, remember that we'll get there soon enough.

- *Stop giving advice.* We know—this is like telling you to turn over the car keys, the checkbook, and the investment portfolio to someone who keeps his money in a piggy bank. But it's important to realize that most of your advice to this point hasn't helped your child get rid of OCD. Do whatever you can to trust this program and your child's desire to be rid of OCD and stick to your role of offering support and reinforcement for progress made against the illness. (See the sidebar on page 104 for some ideas on avoiding giving advice.)

- *Be your child's most loyal cheerleader.* One of your most constructive tasks will be to be supportive of and confident in your child's abilities to do the anti-OCD tasks involved in this program. This means saying "I know it is hard, but you can do this" instead of "Maybe next time" when he's having difficulty.

- *Praise your child for any victory over OCD, no matter how small, but always in terms of the child's satisfaction with the achievement, not as a way of grading performance.* If you say "good job," you're likely to raise your child's anxiety about his or her "performance" against OCD. If you say "pretty neat," you'll reinforce your child's internal sense of accomplishment. Remember, the child's victories over OCD are not being won for your benefit or anyone else's but your child's. When you reinforce the child's positive feelings by saying something like "Cool, I bet it feels good to turn the tables on OCD," you constantly remind your child of how gratifying it is to make progress against OCD, and that is highly motivating.

- *Reinforce other, positive behavior.* OCD seems to get worse the more direct attention it gets. Rather than focusing your attention on your child's OCD obsessions or compulsions as they occur, try training your attention on more pleasant things, such as things that go well that have nothing to do with OCD. Remember, you have a normal child who happens to have OCD. Pay attention to the things that go well and, by not harping about OCD, you'll convey confidence that your child is up to the task of resisting OCD. Also, you'll have a lot more fun. Take a break from OCD and remember all the things that go well with you, with your child, and in your relationship. Call up some memories that make you feel good about yourself and about each other. Remember a few things you're looking forward to that have nothing to do with OCD. Do this both when together and when apart. What we're looking for here is a bit of pleasure and sympathetic understanding about things that have nothing to do with OCD. Besides putting OCD in its rightful place, this will make it easier to be an impartial observer of how OCD operates because you'll have a much better frame of reference by which to see clearly what is and what isn't OCD.

- *Plan to stop helping with rituals, but only at a pace agreed on by all of you according to the program outlined in this book.* If you've been involved in your child's rituals, as so many families are, you'll have to ease your way out of them, just as your child must. But don't plan on doing this abruptly. In fact, don't plan on doing it at all without your child's consent. We'll teach you how to decide when to tackle OCD and when OCD is too tough to tackle. If you need to do this quickly because OCD is too severe—for example, if you are chronically late for work and in danger of losing your job because of your child's OCD—then self-help won't be enough, and you will need to find a therapist to help with structuring cognitive-behavioral treatment that can tackle OCD more quickly. Without a plan that both you and your child have agreed on, you won't have a way to manage the distress that will result from withdrawing your participation in rituals all at once.

- *Use rewards, ceremonies, and notifications to encourage your child.* Rewards and other positive reinforcement from parents cannot be at the center of OCD treatment, because it's what the child, not the parents, does that counts most. The rest of us can provide support, but in the end only the child can turn and face OCD and cease doing rituals. But parents can and should help motivate the child to do the hard work of resisting OCD. For example, spontaneous or planned prizes or treats for individual victories over OCD are a good thing, especially when kids have been subjected to a lot of criticism or punishment for their OCD behavior. They may be particularly useful with very young children. You can also use more symbolic recognition, in the form of planned ceremonies to mark certain milestones against OCD. For example, when a particularly difficult OCD symptom has been vanquished, a trip with friends to the pizza parlor may be in order, not as a reward but rather to celebrate and recognize a job well done. And notification—telling others who need to know of your child's achievements toward getting better—not only will reinforce the child's work directly but also may gain the child support from those who haven't offered it in the past.

> Fifteen-year-old Sam had had OCD for 7 years when he started treatment. He and his parents quickly labeled OCD as OCD, and Sam got to work on building the skills taught in this program. His parents, who were astonished at the enthusiasm Sam showed, went agreeably along with the program, in part because they recognized that all the advice, bribes, punishments, and other things they'd tried had only strained their relationship with Sam. As Sam progressed, his parents began expressing spontaneous joy in Sam's own feelings of pleasure in resisting OCD. They also began to reward his progress, for example, by adding spending money for pleasant activities, such as going to a movie with friends. They also set up "payoffs" that Sam could work toward, not just to motivate him but also to recognize his achievements in resisting OCD. Finally, with Sam's consent, they helped Sam tell his favorite grandmother about OCD, so that she too could understand why Sam had seemed so distant and, in turn, could share in the family's happiness about how treatment was proceeding.

• *Be creative.* Talk to your child about what is and isn't helpful. Try to understand the difference between "can't" and "won't" so that you don't expect the impossible. This may vary from day to day and will certainly vary with different OCD symptoms. Don't confuse OCD with other aspects of your child's behavior, whether good or bad. Be sensitive to your child's age and temperament and trust that he knows what is best for himself, within limits set by his age and propensity to exercise good judgment. Be creative in helping your son think up ways to resist OCD, but stay with the program at all times.

• *Keep your child's developmental stage and relative maturity in mind.* Throughout this book we'll give you ideas for being more heavily involved with each step for younger or less mature kids, but it's important that you use all your knowledge of your child's emotional and mental maturity in deciding when to help and when to give your son or daughter free rein.

• *Be realistic without being pessimistic.* When I talk about getting rid of the child's OCD, I mean getting to the point where no one but the child knows that OCD is still lurking in the background and may pop up from time to time. OCD tends to be

How to Stop Giving Advice

When your child gets lost in a compulsion, cut off the urge to force him to stop or to give unhelpful advice by reminding yourself that . . .

> you wouldn't yell at your daughter to stop coughing if she had a cold.
>
> you wouldn't try to talk your son out of vomiting if he had a stomach virus.
>
> you wouldn't tell your daughter she was letting her basketball team down by not playing with a broken leg.
>
> you wouldn't tell your son that he could take on the local street gang if only he got a little tougher.
>
> you wouldn't insist that your child enter a masters' chess tournament when he's never played the game.
>
> you wouldn't accuse your 8-year-old of disobeying when she was unable to do a calculus problem.

And neither should you harass, punish, or try to reason with a child who is completely stuck in the midst of an attack of OCD. Stop giving advice and start responding with patience and kindness. Stay with the program, and step by step OCD will disappear. To the extent that you do this, your child will begin to treat him- or herself the same way, which will help immeasurably when it comes time for EX/RP.

Instead of saying . . .	Try saying . . .
"It's so stupid to keep doing this!"	"OCD is so hard to deal with, isn't it? It will pass; just let it go as best you can."
"Will you hurry up!"	"Anything I can do to help make it go more easily?"
"Just stop it!"	"Just remember, as with bad weather, OCD always stops. Try to resist as best you can, and when you're ready, we'll go on with what we were doing."
"I can't believe you're doing this again!"	"I'm so sorry you're hurting. This one is pretty hard. Just do the best you can and we'll get there."
"You know the program says you should be doing X, Y, or Z. Maybe you should try a little harder."	"Is there any way I can support you in doing the program?"

a lifelong illness for some people, and it waxes and wanes depending on many different factors. But with the skills imparted in this book, it can be kept under control and is never debilitating. If your child is one of the lucky ones, and there are many, it will go away completely, never to return. When you talk to your child about OCD, talk about eliminating the problems that OCD causes, doing what you can do today to resist OCD, and accepting with kindness and patience those aspects of OCD that will have to wait until tomorrow.

Other Family Members

Family members such as siblings who are either involved with rituals or who don't understand what OCD is need to be educated and become part of the program. When everyone is mixed up with or about OCD, get help from a therapist experienced at disentangling kids and families from OCD.

Therapists, Doctors, and Other Helpers

The best way to use this book may be to work with a therapist who is using our guide for therapists, *OCD in Children and Adolescents: A Cognitive-Behavioral Treatment Manual*. That way you'll be able to work cooperatively from the same program. You can also look to the "How a Therapist Can Help" sections for signals that your child needs expert advice or assistance, but a professional with whom you are already working may very well have ideas about the type and level of involvement that would benefit you. Be sure to ask what the doctor prefers, and be sure that your doctor, too, is working from the program as outlined in our book for professionals.

Teachers and School Staff

It's not uncommon for school performance to slide to some extent before a child with OCD gets successful treatment, especially when the rituals of OCD trap schoolwork. For example, reading and rereading rituals can make it impossible for a child to get homework done. Where OCD interferes with school performance by taking up time, or when rituals directly interfere with school tasks, it's important for school staff to know that your child is struggling with an illness and what that illness entails. Teachers may even become active members of the treatment team, but at the very least you should expect the child with OCD to be treated with kindness and compassion at school, as at home.

Support Groups

Support groups, some of which can be found on the Internet, can be a huge help when any or all of you are frustrated and tired of battling OCD. Even if your child doesn't want to get involved, you might benefit from talking to other parents about what OCD has put them through. See Chapter 4 and the Resources section at the back of the book. If you go this route, though, remember that not everyone will be familiar with the research documenting the effectiveness of this program. So if other parents tout medication as an instant cure, please keep in mind what you read in Chapter 2: that medication can help put OCD in the background but that it's this type of CBT that keeps OCD away for good. A search for a magic pill is a big distraction that will only get in the way of learning the skills you and your child need to learn to get rid of OCD.

Get a Picture of the Whole Program

It's just as important that you have a complete grasp of the whole program, how the steps proceed, and what kind of work is involved as it is that your child does. You'll be providing support and encouragement throughout, so you may need to set your child gently back on track or remind your son or daughter of how well it's going. This program is called a "time-limited" program because it has a distinct beginning and end and is intended to build on itself progressively. So be sure you understand the course from start to finish. If you need to, reread Chapter 4 to get a fuller idea of what the EX/RP form of CBT involves.

The following box gives you a handy reference to what happens at each step and which chapter covers it.

Tips for supporting your child's work during Step 1: *Patience* and *understanding* should be your bywords. Keep in mind that your child will think like a child (or a teenager) during this work, as in other parts of life. Especially in the middle of an OCD attack, kids often have trouble keeping a realistic perspective about obsessions and compulsions. Don't expect to have a rational conversation in the middle of a ritual. Many children are also embarrassed about having OCD and will try to keep it secret, especially if they feel judged or believe disclosure will only lead to demands to stop.

Helping younger kids: Younger children (preschool to elementary school) with OCD will often find the support of a parent essential. This program will help you become a coach for your child and, in that role, you'll be a supporter and an assistant, particularly at the beginning, as your child moves through the program. Once she gets the hang of it, you'll fade out a bit, coming back in to celebrate successes, disentangle yourself from OCD if necessary, and perhaps help with the hardest EX/RP tasks at the end.

Helping teenagers: OCD can wreak havoc with a teenager's natural striving for independence. First, OCD can make the teen dependent on parents in practical terms; for example, by tangling parents and teens up in rituals together. Second, OCD can interfere with the teen's ability to psychologically grow into his true self. The best way to handle this is to acknowledge that OCD is the problem, that being a teenager is just what it is, normal, and that the solution to getting rid of OCD is to follow the

The Program Steps at a Glance

Step 1 (this chapter): Education about OCD and its treatment.

Goals: (1) Make sure everyone knows that OCD, not the child, is the problem; (2) define OCD as a neurobehavioral illness; (3) get everyone on the child's side; and (4) make sure everyone understands how the treatment works. (*Weeks 1–2*)

Step 2 (Chapter 6): Beginning to map OCD and introducing the "toolkit."

Goals: (1) The child learns how to talk to himself and others about OCD; (2) the idea of "bossing back" OCD and how to take it at the child's own constructive pace is introduced. (*Weeks 1–2*)

Step 3 (Chapter 7): Finishing mapping OCD.

Goals: (1) The child uses her list of symptoms to sketch out a plan of attack; (2) the child keeps her thoughts straight about OCD. (*Weeks 1–2*)

Step 4 (Chapter 8): Finishing the toolkit.

Goals: (1) The child uses the map of OCD to test picking targets for EX/RP from the work zone; (2) the child practices EX/RP using the toolkit as a "dress rehearsal" for taking on OCD for real. (*Weeks 1–2*)

Step 5 (Chapter 9): Beginning to resist OCD.

Goals: (1) The child undertakes the first battles with OCD; (2) the family figures out how allies (family members) are involved (or not) with OCD and, if they are, begins to extricate them from OCD's grasp. (*Weeks 3–5*)

Note: The pace for the rest of the program will vary with different children, but the whole program should take about 3 months and no more than 5. If more than 3 months are needed, they will be added during Steps 6–8.

Step 6 (Chapter 10): Fighting back against OCD in earnest.

Goals: (1) The child continues exposure and response prevention; (2) the family plans ceremonies and rewards to celebrate victories. (*Weeks 6–10*)

Step 7 (Chapter 11): Eliminating OCD everywhere.

Goals: (1) Progress review; (2) plateaus are addressed; (3) harder EX/RP tasks are chosen; (4) the child selects a task for parents. (*Weeks 6–10*)

Step 8 (Chapter 12): Getting along without OCD.

Goal: (1) Relapse prevention. (*Weeks 11–12*)

program outlined in this book. If this proves impossible because of teen–parent "issues," then you'll need a therapist to help move things forward.

How a therapist can help: If you get stuck and can't get unstuck, find a trained mental health professional with experience using CBT for OCD.

Give OCD a Funny Nickname or Learn to Call It by Its Medical Name

You can help your child with this task, but be careful not to choose a nickname that demonizes OCD. The younger the child, the less able she may be to tolerate anxiety. A nickname that doesn't provoke a smile but instead scares the child should be avoided. We want to bring OCD down in size, not inflate it. If your child wants to choose a rather scary or threatening name, steer him or her in a more lighthearted direction: Instead of "Killer," suggest "Mr. Stupid." Rather than "Dr. Death," how about "Dodohead"? Also, just talking this way about OCD can make OCD "get upset." If this happens, just remember to go easy. A light, kind hand is always better than pushing through the program.

When you start to practice referring to OCD as a third party in the room, say things like "What's up with OCD today?" and "How's Stinky treating you?" and "Can you give me an example of how you beat OCD today?" and "OCD's up to its old tricks, huh?"

Your goal is to bring an attitude of kindness and generosity of heart to developing a close understanding of OCD and how to get rid of it. Without the ability to accept where you are rather than where you wish you were and to treat each other with kindness, it's very hard to pay close attention to what is happening with OCD, which is an absolute prerequisite to implementing the rest of the program. Remember, there are no grades here, just everyone together trying to end the suffering that OCD causes and, with OCD gone, to bring about the ordinary happiness of a life lived reasonably well.

You can do a lot to set the appropriate tone here, not just in this homework session but in general. Make sure your child knows you're taking a new attitude toward OCD, one that says it's not to be taken too seriously, that the child is in charge and everyone now knows it. Laugh gently about OCD as much as you can, but don't force it. As you know, kids can spot a phony a mile away, and there is a very slippery slope between laughing with the child about OCD and making the child with OCD the butt of a joke. Matt's mom, Sarah, started out right, saying to 10-year-old Matt, "Old Numero is such a pain, keeping you stuck with all that counting, isn't he? I mean, what does he think you are, a calculator?" This kind of banter distracted Matt from feeling bad about keeping his mother waiting while he retraced his steps several times to count the tiles on the floor on his way out. But then Sarah went too far without realizing it: "I mean, who needs to count stuff like that? What a dumb waste of time!" It was a subtle shift, and totally unintentional, but when she stopped attributing Matt's actions to OCD, her son started feeling that he was responsible for this "dumb waste of time" and withdrew into a shamed silence, in which OCD made him feel like the only way out of the unpleasant feelings was to count in his head. Keep your joking in the third person, as well as simple and short; it's too easy to take a wrong turn if you go on and on.

Start Noticing Where OCD Wins and Where Your Child Wins

As you are likely involved in or at least can observe many of your child's rituals, you can help the child notice when OCD is winning and when the child is winning. This is also your opportunity to establish a new tone in talking to your child about OCD. With a neutral tone of voice, simply point out gently and uncritically, "I guess OCD won that time," or "Looks you beat Old Germy that time, didn't you?" As a general rule, you can tell what help to give your child by listening to his questions and providing only those answers that reflect what the child wants to know and that are consistent with the program.

Helping younger kids: Pointing out where OCD wins or loses at the time, using OCD's new nickname, will help young children start to think of OCD as something separate from themselves, which is often difficult because they haven't developed much insight yet. It can also help them see OCD in a more humorous light and thus minimize anxiety.

Helping teenagers: Because parental inquiries are often seen by teens as just "rubbing it in," it may be best to stick to "How's OCD behaving?" When your teen does want to talk, be thankful and restrict yourself to clarifying his thoughts, not giving advice other than to reinforce the need to follow the program.

Taking Stock

Help your child focus on successes and steer her away from viewing anything as a failure or defeat. Make completing the scale and graph on pages 95–96 fun, like any art project. Make sure you find a place to keep your graph throughout the program if you've copied it rather than filling it in right in the book. You'll be comparing the graph drawn each week so that your child can see his or her steady progress. If your child finds writing a chore rather than an aid, volunteer to be his scribe.

6

Step 2: Talking Back to OCD

John is a normal 15-year-old who happens to have OCD. He likes school but likes music and his friends better. Most of all, he can't wait until he gets his driver's license, something his parents aren't so sure about. John, who has had OCD for many years, makes it quite clear that he hates it. Even more, he hates the feeling that he can't do anything about it. He's taken different medications, some of which have been a bit helpful, but he doesn't like the side effects or even the idea of taking medicine. John's parents feel bad that problems with OCD have made everyone unhappy, including John's younger sister, Rebecca, who often feels ignored because so much of the family's life turns on coping with OCD.

John's mother read about our program in the book for therapists (*OCD in Children and Adolescents*) and then told John about it. After hesitating at first, John took a look at the book, too, and pretty quickly decided to call OCD by its medical name. He also told his parents for the first time how much he hated OCD and how it made him feel stupid inside. John's honesty broke the ice, and the family started talking about how they might put the program to work for their family. For the first time in a long time, they all felt that there was hope for beating OCD, especially now that they were treating it the way it should be treated—as an illness separate from John.

John especially liked the fact that, in this program, his parents were supposed to stop giving him advice about how to deal with OCD. His parents especially liked the idea that John was going to be responsible for skillfully managing his relationship to OCD. Of course, John and his parents and sister liked knowing that he had a good shot at beating OCD.

Everyone agreed that they'd give it a try and seek out a CBT therapist only if they couldn't make a go of it. They did, and 3 months later, John was mostly free of OCD.

In Step 1 you gave OCD a name of its own, and if all went well, everyone in the family now gets the idea that OCD is not Shelly or Eric or Dan. OCD is not *you*. It's Germy, Mr. Stupid, Dodohead—or just an illness with its own name, OCD. The thoughts, urges, images—whatever pops up when OCD hiccups—have no real meaning; they are just brain hiccups that you can learn to ignore safely. When you do so, OCD will stop hiccupping.

In Step 2 you'll start to talk back to Germy or OCD. But you'll still be taking it slowly. Steps 1 and 2 are all about testing the water so you see how strong you already are and so your parents understand how to play their part without getting in your way. For now, practice being patient with yourself about OCD. Resist as best you can, and don't blame yourself when OCD makes you feel like you have to do rituals. Jumping off the high board before you can swim is not a good idea. For now, just remember that rituals are part of OCD, not something that has real meaning and purpose for you. You'll still have OCD to deal with, but you won't be lost in it anymore, and that's a big step forward.

We were really excited when we first saw the doctor and started on the program, but then I got ahead of myself and tried to touch a toilet seat at school and not wash before I was ready. Boy, was that a mistake. I had a really bad time with OCD and ended up not getting to class on time, it took so long to wash. The good news is a few weeks later I was ready and it went fine—actually a little easier than I ever thought it would be.

—Nora, age 14

My dad got real mad at me when I told him and my mom some of the ways I could resist OCD already. He thought if I could stop one thing, I could stop all of it, but Mom convinced him it's important to take it one step at a time. It makes it a lot easier to keep my eye on OCD when they're on my side and not fighting.

—Adam, age 11

Just knowing OCD as OCD, even while you still do rituals or avoid the things OCD makes you afraid of, is power—real power that means you aren't simply obeying OCD's orders anymore. This power prepares you to take a closer look at OCD. To get a clearer view of what this illness is really like, you're going to practice watching OCD, learning its quirks and schemes, for the next week or two. How does it operate and how does it affect your life? Does OCD mind your business mostly at home or at school? Does it like to keep you checking things over and over? Or does it insist on a certain strict routine at mealtime, bedtime, or bathtime? In the same way you might scout the opposition before a basketball game, getting to know the characteristics of OCD will help you beat it.

In Step 2 you'll also be getting to know yourself at the same time as you're getting to know OCD. Can you push yourself to be a little bolder with OCD? When does talking back to OCD just feel too dangerous? Where do you win sometimes and lose sometimes with OCD? Where is OCD not a problem? Where is it impossible to resist?

The Game Plan for Step 2

Follow the directions under "Get Ready"; you'll start by looking back at what you did in Step 1. Then spend about a week following the instructions in this chapter, putting in about 30 to 60 minutes every day. (You'll also be adding in Steps 3 and 4 before the week is up, but don't worry about that now. Keep checking off the fact that you've done your homework each day, using the "Getting Stronger Every Day" chart that you should have posted wherever you'll see it easily and often.) Keep working together as a family and get a therapist's help if you need it. Here are a few important tips for success:

- *Do your homework.* OCD is an illness, and it won't get better unless you work at it. Just like a patient with diabetes who has to watch diet and exercise, you have to retrain your brain so it will stop hiccupping. If you skimp on practice, you won't get very good at resisting OCD, and having OCD is not good for your growing brain. So take the work seriously, but have some fun while doing it. OCD really is goofy, and you can enjoy learning to resist the same way you enjoy going on a roller coaster or riding fast on your bike.
- *Ask for support when you need it.* You're just getting started, and it's perfectly normal to feel like you need a boost or some reassurance that you're doing the right thing. Whenever that happens, use your OCD nickname to alert your parents: "Mr. Stupid is really bugging me today, Mom. Would you watch TV with me?" "Germy seems to be all over the place today, Dad. Can we play catch for a while?"
- *Feel comfortable that you've reached the goals for this step before moving on to the next step.* Never skip the "Taking Stock" wrap-up at the end of each step! If you've gotten stuck, talk to a therapist.

It took me 2 weeks just to feel OK calling OCD Mr. Pottymouth in my head. I was really afraid those bad thoughts meant I was going to go to hell. That's what I learned at church about nasty thoughts, and it took time for me to realize they weren't my thoughts but belonged to Mr. Pottymouth. He's just a brain hiccup. God wants me to get well.

—Darren, age 12

- *Remind yourself of what you do well.* Don't worry about any trouble you had with Step 1, and don't get down on yourself if you think you didn't get very far. Concentrate on your successes. Whatever you accomplished, it's a real success and will make a difference. So give yourself a big pat on the back and continue what you did in Step 1 while you add Step 2. Also, remember what else you did last week for which you deserve a few points: Solve a really tough math problem? Play Legos with your little sister when you would rather have played football? Finish your book report book ahead of time? Take your brother to soccer practice so your mom could finish that report she brought home from work? All of this is you, and you deserve a big round of applause.

Get Ready

Tear out the summary sheet for Step 2 from the back of this book or make a copy of it and stick it on your refrigerator, your bathroom mirror, your closet door, or wherever you're likely to see it most often.

Before you get going on the tasks for Step 2, make sure the nickname you came up with for OCD in Step 1 (or just its medical name if that's what you chose) is working for you. The nickname you chose should make you feel hopeful and a little more in charge of OCD than you did before. It especially should make it easier to see OCD as an illness different from you—not so "sticky." But some kids hate OCD so much that they naturally choose a name they would imagine belonging to a monster or a bully. Unfortunately, calling OCD something like "Killer" or "Devil" sometimes puffs OCD up. We want to shrink OCD back to its true size—small and manageable. So if your nickname for OCD made you feel worried, scared, or uncomfortable, try the following solutions.

- If your nickname for OCD has made you feel more helpless than ever, or if you just want another, "easier" name, try a sillier, less nasty one. One girl we know chose Washerman, another picked Oink, and then there was Dirtball, Mr.

Nasty, Bill, and Terrible Trouble (TT). One boy called OCD Mr. Adams after a teacher who didn't understand and repeatedly punished him for OCD.

- If your nickname for OCD made OCD mad, but you still were able to resist doing rituals as much as before and it wasn't too upsetting, that's fine. It'll get better.

- If your nickname made OCD mad and you found it harder than ever to resist OCD, you probably found yourself arguing with yourself. If you try not to think about something, you just think about it more. The goal of the exercise is to reveal OCD as impersonal. If the nickname you chose personalizes OCD even more, choose another nickname that has a bit more relaxed humor. Try out the new name and see if it makes it easier to keep OCD at a distance. If the whole nickname idea doesn't seem to be working, just use the term OCD. That's what it is anyway. When OCD shows up, simply note that OCD is present. Say "Hi, OCD" as though it is another person in the room and go on about your business. The real point is not the name itself but to put OCD outside yourself so you don't get lost in it anymore. Then you can learn OCD's tricks and get it to stop hiccupping.

I called OCD "Killer" because it used to kill me to have to do all those rituals, but at first it was too scary. I stuck with it, though, because my therapist told me a story about a little dog with arthritis named Killer who wouldn't hurt a flea. That made me laugh and helped me learn to laugh at OCD, too.

—Alex, age 8

I thought the idea of giving OCD a nickname was good for younger kids, but not for me. I just called it OCD. Talking to OCD like it was a person in the room and laughing a bit about it was really helpful, though I must admit OCD didn't like the idea much.

—Lakisha, age 15

I called OCD David after this kid who picks on me 'cause of my rituals. David is not a friend to me and neither is OCD, though I suppose there's hope for David. That's funny.

—Corey, age 12

When I first tried to call OCD by its medical name, I got scared because I didn't like the idea of being sick. Then I began to be able to watch OCD and was able to see that what OCD said wasn't really what I believed. OCD was more like the weather, bad sometimes, not so bad other times,

*and I just had to deal with it. Now when I call OCD by its name, it's like
talking to my dermatologist about acne. Kind of a pain—I wish I didn't
have it—but not the same thing as me.*

—Alice, age 13

How a therapist can help: If things don't go smoothly at Step 2, keep in mind
that a therapist can help you figure out where things went wrong. A therapist can
also help you practice, give you examples from all the other kids he's treated, and
come up with strategies that will work for your particular family. Don't hesitate to
ask for help or support. You don't want to let yourself get discouraged so early in
the program.

Get Going

Make OCD the Problem

Calling OCD by its own name has already set you well on your way to Goal 1, making OCD, not you or your family, the problem. Now you'll show yourself without a
doubt that OCD is *not* you but something separate by using your mind to see OCD as
something that pops up uninvited and makes you unhappy.

Start thinking about the following questions. You can talk them over with Mom
or Dad or just review them on your own. You don't have to write down your
answers, but if it feels like it might help, go ahead and do so. Be sure to use the
nickname you've given OCD in the questions.

- How has OCD bossed you around over the last few days?
- How does OCD mess things up for you at home? At school? With your friends?
- How have you said "no" to OCD?
- Can you give an example of how you successfully resisted OCD over the last
  few days?
- When you triumphed over OCD, how did it feel? What did you say to your-
  self?
- Who helps you boss OCD back?
- How would the person you admire most boss OCD around?
- Who do you most want to know about your success in getting rid of OCD?
- What will your life without OCD look like?

There's no "right" answer to these questions. The answers just help you think
more and more about OCD as something "out there" and not in your head. If you

ask yourself these questions a few more days into Step 2, you can compare your answers with the earlier ones and see where your successes as well as problems have been. But even more important, the simple act of working these questions into conversations with yourself and with your parents is terrific practice in making OCD an outsider. Kids who have been waging their own internal battles with OCD for some time, as most do, end up feeling as if their minds are thoroughly entangled with the illness. Just getting OCD out in the open and talking about it as an illness goes a long way toward leading you out of the maze that OCD has created. Many kids, in fact, end up talking over these questions and their answers with their parents every couple of days, not as homework but because they represent one way out of the trap set by OCD. As with so many other things, the reward lies in the practice!

Start to Map OCD

Your answers to the previous questions gave you some important information about what OCD tries to get you to do and when and where it succeeds in getting you to do it. They also show you where OCD isn't around at all and, when it is, when you've been able to tell it to jump in the lake. In this second part of Step 2, you're going to use this information to draw a map (in chart form) that shows where you rule and, for the time being, where OCD still runs your life. This "map," which you'll fill in over the next week and then keep drawing for the rest of the program, will be a key tool in helping you come up with a successful battle plan against OCD.

Let's look a little more closely at how OCD operates. Maybe OCD makes you feel terrified that your mother is going to catch germs from you and get sick, so you feel like you have to wash a lot. Or perhaps OCD makes you feel like things have to be balanced between left and right, so you might spend a lot of time getting things evened up or arranged in a certain way. These examples describe two of the more common types of OCD, and many kids have both. In the first kind, a normal feeling (a worry about someone you love getting sick) gets exaggerated; it's way bigger than what you'd feel about the real risk that your mother will get sick, and it just doesn't make a whole lot of sense. The second is a need to have things "just so," and it often feels like an itch that won't go away, no matter how hard or how long you scratch. In both cases, OCD has a bad deal to offer you: Perform certain rituals and your fear about your mom or your urge to make things symmetrical will go away. It's a bad deal because what it doesn't tell you is that the bad feelings or fears will go away only for a while. Taking this deal, as you know, traps you in a vicious circle that starts with a trigger (seeing your mom or putting on your socks, for example) or just starts out of nowhere, which leads to an obsession (your mom will catch your germs and get sick, or getting your socks even is crucial), which feels like it will go away only if you obey a compulsion (wash your hands to rid them of germs or straighten your socks over and over until the feeling that you're germy or your socks aren't even goes away). You know all about this cycle, from reading Chapter 2 of this book and from your own experience.

As you continue to talk back to OCD this week, using your special nickname for it, try to think of each run-in with OCD as having those three parts—trigger, obsession, compulsion (keeping in mind that for some OCD "hiccups" there is no trigger; the hiccups just show up). Ask yourself these questions, and put your answers in your own words (it's not a test!):

- What triggered OCD? Or did it just pop up out of nowhere?
- What is the obsession like?
- What thoughts and feelings make it an obsession as compared with normal (not OCD) worries or urges?
- What is a compulsion like?
- How long does the obsession last if you do the rituals? How long when you don't do the rituals?
- Does how you talk to yourself while OCD is around have any impact on obsessions or compulsions?
- Does talking about OCD as an illness help you not get lost in OCD? Does this make it easier to resist doing rituals?

Thinking in this way so you get to know the triggers, obsessions, and compulsions that define OCD for you will help you do the work of Steps 3 and 4, as well as this step. Right now, your main goal is to start figuring out how OCD works. Start by thinking about the situations in which you have the types of OCD thoughts and feelings you just identified. Using the following form (you can make copies), see if you can write down five to eight symptoms (hiccups) of OCD that cause you trouble. If you have more than one flavor of OCD, it may help to group them into one of these types: washing, checking, ordering or arranging, counting or repeating, moral or religious OCD, and hoarding. List the triggering situation if there is one, the obsession, and the ritual. For now, don't worry about the temperature (Temp.) column. We'll introduce that tool for ranking OCD from "hard-" to "easy-to-resist" in a moment. Just try to include some easy-to-resist OCD symptoms, some middle-sized ones, and one or two really hard-to-resist symptoms. If the hardest are too hard, meaning that just thinking about them sets OCD off, stick to the easier ones. If there are some that you can't talk about with anyone, just put them down as "OCD X" and so on. That puts a marker in place so that at the right time you can

Your Symptoms (Hiccups): Mapping OCD

Action/situation/trigger (if any)	Obsession	Compulsion	Temp. (1–10)

Your Symptoms (Hiccups): Mapping OCD
Example

Action/situation/trigger (if any)	Obsession	Compulsion	Temp. (1–10)
Touching doorknobs	"I'll get people's germs and get sick."	Use shirt, tissue, or coat to hold doorknobs.	
Using friend's bathroom	"I'll get their family's germs and make my family sick."	Avoid visiting for long enough to need the bathroom.	
Touching my mouth with my fingers	"I'll get sick and die from germs on my hands."	Wash hands every time my fingers touch my mouth.	
Petting the dog	"The dog's germs will spread and make everyone sick."	Pet dog with gloves on or wash hands 5 times.	
Touching toilet	"I'll get germy and make Mom sick."	Avoid touching toilet or wash hands 5 times.	
Touching bathroom sink	Same	Avoid touching sink or wash hands 5 times.	
Getting dressed for school	"I have to make sure my socks are evened up."	Even up socks over and over until they feel right. Ask Mom whether they look straight.	
Same	"My watch has to be right in the middle of my wrist."	Don't wear watch or adjust it on my wrist till it looks right.	

fill in the needed information. And it tells OCD that you're doing what you need to without doing what is impossible at this point. Don't try to think of every single way that OCD bosses you around; just list several big-ticket examples of easy, medium, and impossible to resist for now.

Starting with your list of what OCD does and using the answers you gave under "Make OCD the Problem," you're now going to think more carefully about the dividing line between your life with OCD and your life without it. You probably had some wins and some losses last week, like most other kids. Right now, if you drew a picture showing where you win and where OCD wins on an average day, you'd get something like this:

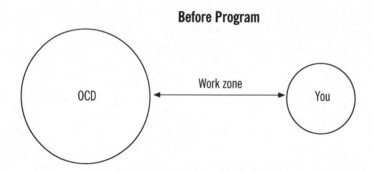

Before Program

The bigger circle represents OCD's territory—where OCD always wins and has pretty much complete control over your life. The smaller circle represents your territory—where you can count on winning and having total control. For example, if you were to touch a glass and hug your mom, OCD might be nowhere to be seen, since this isn't a big deal for you—though it might be for another youngster with OCD. However, if you were to touch a toilet seat, OCD might make you feel like you had to wash many times before you could hug your mom. Here OCD controls everything, because, for the time being, you don't have the skills to do the opposite of what OCD wants.

Now notice the space in between the two circles. We call this the *work zone*; it's where you win some of the time and OCD wins some of the time—like maybe when you want to hug Mom after touching the dog or cat. Sometimes you can do it without washing; sometimes you can't. We call this the work zone because you're going to work at claiming this "land" for yourself. The basic idea, which is really what makes this program work, is that it's easier to turn partial success into 100% success than to try to turn failure (where OCD always wins) to 100% successful resistance.

In this program, you'll never be asked to do the impossible. When you decide the time is right not to cooperate with OCD, you will be in the work zone, which is where you already know how to win. You just need to do it more often until you've taken back that territory from OCD. As you get to know OCD over the next few weeks, you'll get very good at identifying the triggers, obsessions, and compulsions that fall into the work zone, so you can start working toward taking control over them. As you go along, the picture or map of your OCD will begin to look more and more like this:

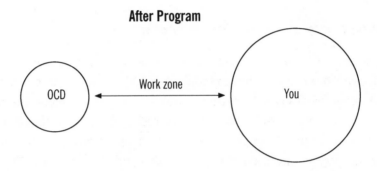

After Program

OCD ←— Work zone —→ You

Territory claimed by OCD becomes yours again as you learn more about OCD, develop new skills and strategies, gain confidence in yourself, and learn that, in fact, you can resist OCD successfully to the point that your brain no longer hiccups.

Angela, age 9, started to cry when she saw the map. She has mild OCD, and it just didn't seem to her that OCD took up as much space as the map showed. When she saw the "before" diagram, she got really worried that OCD would grow, but we talked about how working to see OCD clearly is a way to stop getting lost in thoughts and worries. Using her nickname (Goofy Thinking, or GT for short) to talk about it, we drew a more accurate diagram that made the OCD circle smaller. That was all it took to make things right.

I got the idea of the work zone right away, but it was hard to see how I could take control of things that were higher up [harder, under OCD's control]. When I told my mom how worried I was about this, she reminded me to read through the rest of the book. When I did, I saw how, as you work through the program, the work zone gradually takes over all the territory that used to be OCD's, until there's no OCD left. Hard stuff gets easier with practice. Like you're going up a ladder, the work zone moves up, and like magic, hard stuff isn't so hard anymore. After that, I kept the book around and referred to it a lot whenever I felt stuck or afraid that I wasn't going to get better.

—Howard, age 17

Keep in mind that even using a nickname and poking fun at OCD may seem kind of frightening at first, especially if it gets OCD going. If you feel stuck, ask your parents for a little moral support or talk to your therapist.

Get to Know the Fear Thermometer

As you and your parents know all too well, some pretty uncomfortable feelings come with obsessions. These feelings can be so hard to tolerate that many kids can't bring themselves to resist OCD at all. If you're among the many kids who come down hard on themselves for not resisting, try to remember this: Whether simple (fear of germs) or complex (fear that you might hurt someone), fear is the strongest signal the brain ever sends. And for good reason. Fear is the brain's alarm system. If we don't listen to its danger warnings, we can end up in big trouble. OCD is counting on the fact that you'll have a hard time ignoring those alarm bells. So don't beat yourself up if you find fear (or other bad feelings, such as disgust or "just so" feelings, that go with OCD) hard to resist; that's the way the brain is supposed to work. You're about to meet a tool that will help you tone down the siren so you can get beyond fear and beat OCD, a little baby step at a time.

This is what we call a fear thermometer. It will help you rank your fears so you can see exactly where you will be able to win against OCD. It's important for you to pick your own fights with OCD. The fear thermometer will help you do it so that you, not OCD, emerge the winner. Although we call it the fear thermometer, it

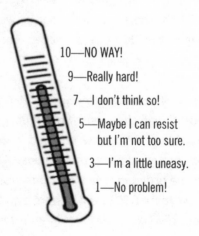

10—NO WAY!

9—Really hard!

7—I don't think so!

5—Maybe I can resist
but I'm not too sure.

3—I'm a little uneasy.

1—No problem!

really measures all the uncomfortable feelings that go along with OCD, so don't worry if your particular OCD symptoms involve urges or images or "just so" feelings. The fear thermometer will work fine for them, too.

Let's start by not thinking of OCD at all. Instead, think of the lowest temperature, 1, on the thermometer as the easiest, least scary thing you ever have to do—say, watching your favorite funny TV show or eating your favorite flavor of ice cream. Think of the highest temperature, 10, as the scariest thing you can imagine. One 8-year-old girl we know said this would be getting lost at the state fair. An 11-year-old boy said a 10 for him would be getting stuck in someone's basement with the lights out, just like in the scary movie he just saw. For a 16-year-old, obviously, a 10 would be quite different. A high school student who had just gotten her driver's license said it was driving on the freeway at rush hour. With a bit of help in understanding how it works, she reconsidered and decided this would be a 7 and a bad wreck in those conditions would be a 10.

How easy would it be for you to stay cool in your own personal 1 situation? How about your personal 10? They're very different, aren't they? That's why we don't ask you to do the hard stuff until it gets easy.

Now apply the fear thermometer to OCD as it affects you. Take your list of five to eight symptoms from "Start to Map OCD" and try to figure out where you'd rank them on the fear thermometer. Imagine you're in the situation that triggers OCD so that the obsessions get going, but you don't do the rituals to make them stop. Put differently, use the fear thermometer to grade the ease with which you can resist doing what OCD tells you to do. Or put even another way, use it to rate how hard it would be to break the rules that OCD sets. Is each one a "No problem!" kind of OCD, a "NO WAY!" kind of OCD, or something in between?

Now list the OCD symptoms that bother you on a new sheet of paper, from hardest to easiest to resist. Try to include some easy (1–3), medium (4–7), and hard (8–10) ones on your list. Examples of the two charts are on the next two pages.

Did you list any 2s or 3s? These would be the situations where you can resist your compulsions more than half the time. This is your work zone, and this is where you'll start fighting OCD, because it's much easier to win here than higher up on the thermometer. If you can do more to resist OCD here, do so, but we're not ready to start formal practice yet. For now, and through Steps 3 and 4, you're going to continue scouting OCD by recording information about the obsessions that OCD brings up and how hard it is to resist compulsions when they do come up. Keep doing your best to resist, but don't blame yourself when you can't. You're not expected to be all that successful for the time being, but you'll get there soon. The task now is to get a clear view of the work zone and the OCD "hiccups" just above it.

Your Symptoms (Hiccups): Mapping OCD
Example

Action/situation/trigger (if any)	Obsession	Compulsion	Temp. (1–10)
Touching doorknobs	"I'll get people's germs and get sick."	Use shirt, tissue, or coat to hold doorknobs.	6
Using friend's bathroom	"I'll get their family's germs and make my family sick."	Avoid visiting for long enough to need the bathroom.	8
Touching my mouth with my fingers	"I'll get sick and die from germs on my hands."	Wash hands every time my fingers touch my mouth.	6
Petting the dog	"The dog's germs will spread and make everyone sick."	Pet dog with gloves on or wash hands 5 times.	3–4
Touching toilet	"I'll get germy and make Mom sick."	Avoid touching toilet or wash hands 5 times.	10
Touching bathroom sink	Same	Avoid touching sink or wash hands 5 times.	1–2
Getting dressed for school	"I have to make sure my socks are evened up."	Even up socks over and over until they feel right. Ask Mom whether they look straight.	5
Same	"My watch has to be right in the middle of my wrist."	Don't wear watch or adjust it on my wrist till it looks right.	1–2

Your Symptoms (Hiccups): Mapping OCD
Example: Hardest to Easiest

Action/situation/trigger (if any)	Obsession	Compulsion	Temp. (1–10)
Touching toilet	"I'll get germy and make Mom sick."	Avoid touching toilet or wash hands 5 times.	10
Using friend's bathroom	"I'll get their family's germs and make my family sick."	Avoid visiting for long enough to need the bathroom.	8
Touching my mouth with my fingers	"I'll get sick and die from germs on my hands."	Wash hands every time my fingers touch my mouth.	6
Touching doorknobs	"I'll get people's germs and get sick."	Use shirt, tissue, or coat to hold doorknobs.	6
Getting dressed for school	"I have to make sure my socks are evened up."	Even up socks over and over until they feel right. Ask Mom whether they look straight.	5
Petting the dog	"The dog's germs will spread and make everyone sick."	Pet dog with gloves on or wash hands 5 times.	3–4
Walking by dog after shower	"The dog's germs will spread and make everyone sick."	Don't walk within 6 feet of the dog.	1–2
Getting dressed for school	"My watch has to be right in the middle of my wrist."	Don't wear watch or adjust it on my wrist till it looks right.	1–2

For the next week, add to your symptom list whenever you can, jotting down the number on the fear thermometer that you think represents how easy or hard it is to resist compulsions in that situation. Be creative. It may be that not washing your hands at all is a 10 but that cutting down on the repetitions by one (if you count), doing repetitions out of order (if you have to wash in a certain way), or just cutting down on time (say 8 rather than 10 minutes) would get a lower fear thermometer rating. If so, put that down. The key is to play with the idea that you can grade OCD symptoms by the difficulty you have in triggering OCD on purpose and then not doing the rituals.

How a therapist can help: When OCD is very complicated, and triggers, obsessions, and mental rituals are very hard to sort out, having a therapist to help define what's what can be very helpful.

> *Step 2 was tough for me. I got the idea pretty quickly, but what was hard was not to get going on fighting OCD. All this "go slow" stuff was frustrating me and making me mad until I realized that, just by doing the best I could, 4s were becoming 3s and 3s were becoming 2s and a few little things just went away. The big stuff didn't change at all, though. I think that just knowing that OCD is OCD and talking to myself about it differently has also helped.*
>
> *—Omar, age 14*

> *I like drawing, so the fear thermometer was fun. I put faces next to the numbers, then I drew in the names of my girlfriends or girls I don't like so much. My mom had to help get me back on track when we got to OCD. It isn't really a game, she said; it's about making your brain stop hiccupping. After that, I got more serious.*
>
> *—Angel, age 9*

> *This is really, really, really boring. I hate it, and besides, I have enough homework. That's what I said when my dad asked me to talk to him about how I was doing with the program. Actually, I hadn't done it. Mostly, I do my rituals as quick as I can so I can go skateboarding. Dad understood, but he was still pretty tough about needing to get to work. He's right, of course. I hate having to do this OCD stuff. Anyway, he said, since it's like another chore, he'd buy me a new CD or front me the rent for a movie each week if I did my program homework. If I skip it, though, I'm in trouble. He's pretty cool, my dad, so I did it to humor him: not!*
>
> *—Albert, age 15*

Taking Stock

Finish up this step by completing the OCD scale at the end of Step 1. Then, also as you did at the end of Step 1, plot your answers on the graph on page 96. Remember, there are no "wrong" answers here. The point is just to see how things are going and to feel good about what you accomplish. That's why you're using the "Getting Stronger Every Day" chart to show that you're doing the homework. That's all that matters right now.

When you finish Steps 1 and 2, ask yourself how you feel about OCD now that you've learned to think about it differently. Though OCD undoubtedly still has you doing rituals, you shouldn't feel as bad about that as before. Now you can watch OCD with some understanding rather than feeling plain old helpless or ashamed. Does OCD seem at all easier to resist, harder to resist, or the same? You probably can't yet truly resist OCD, but that won't be true for long. Does your new knowledge about OCD make it easier to relax and be kinder to yourself when you still have to do what OCD says? If not, maybe you don't truly believe OCD is just a brain hiccup. If that's the case, is it possible that you're being too hard on yourself about OCD?

What about family members or friends? Do they now understand OCD the way you do?

Understand that it's the rare person who makes all that much headway against OCD after the first couple of steps. It's later in the program, when your skills really start to mount, that you start beating OCD big time. If you've put a checkmark on your chart for doing the homework for Steps 1 and 2 for the whole first week (or a little more, depending on exactly when you added Step 2), give yourself a big round of applause and share your pride in this accomplishment with your parents and/or therapist. If you haven't done your homework every day, you need to ask yourself whether you are really committed to taking care of yourself or whether you'd rather just put up with OCD than do the hard work necessary to get rid of it. If you haven't really committed to the program, do so now. If you have, and the program seems like it is just too hard to do on your own, you may be one of the many young persons who really needs a skilled CBT therapist. Suggestions for how to find one are at the back of the book.

Step 2: Instructions for Parents

The Game Plan for Step 2

For parents, doing your part in Step 2 means support, support, and—just when you think you've exhausted your reserves—more support. Reread the section on the parents' role in Step 1 whenever you get frustrated with the way things are going—or not going—or whenever you find yourself slipping back into unskillful ways of coping with OCD. Some parents find it helpful to reread those guidelines regularly, say, a couple of times a week, or at least before starting each new step. We'll give tips on how you can help your child with specific tasks as we work through Step 2.

> *Sam and I used to fight all the time about OCD. The last few days I just ask him how OCD is doing. He seems happier now that I'm not riding him about the impossible.*
>
> *—Molly, mother of 11-year-old Sam*

> *Junior and I were best buddies until OCD came between us. Getting us all on the same page has made me realize that this was as much my ignorance as his. It'll take a while to make it better, but I can already see it happening.*
>
> *—Bill, father of 9-year-old Junior*

> *I can remember when Javier was a little boy, before OCD ate up his life. OCD is still the same, but now we all remember what it was like before OCD and have hope that we can get back there again.*
>
> *—Maria, mother of 15-year-old Javier*

As a rabbi, I suppose I should have known the power of giving something its true name, but the change in our family and especially in our son, David, that came about just through labeling OCD an illness has been nothing short of remarkable.
—Abraham, father of 12-year-old David

Here are a couple of important tips for success with this step:

• *Don't hesitate to give your child support.* When your child gives you a signal that she needs extra help, focus on being supportive, reassuring her with kindness and comfort without making a big deal about OCD: "Yeah, I know it's tough, but you're OK." "Old Fussbudget is a real pain, isn't he?" "Just remember it's OCD talking, honey, and you'll be fine. Do the best you can, and don't blame yourself. We're just getting started."

• *Don't be afraid to talk about whether behavior is a "can't" or a "won't."* Sometimes it's tempting to use OCD as an excuse to get out of behaving appropriately. Lots of times it is hard to tell. If you find yourselves unable to tell whether problem behavior is being caused by OCD or just "kids being kids," use your child's nickname for OCD and ask if the behavior in question is related to OCD. Problem behavior is a "won't," whereas OCD at this point in the program is a "can't." We'll talk more about solving the "can't" versus "won't" problem later in the book (see page 222 for more information on managing problem behavior). For now, if it looks like OCD, it is OCD. If it clearly doesn't, do what's appropriate.

Get Ready

As a parent of a child with OCD, it's your job during this review to give your child gentle nudges toward the insights that Step 1 should have made possible. Don't try to lead your child by the hand; do offer questions that encourage the child to look at his thoughts and feelings: "How did OCD make you feel?" "What was the first thing you thought of when OCD showed up?" "What did you think about this later?" Model the attitude that you want your child to adopt by using the child's chosen nickname for OCD whenever you mention OCD: "How did OCD react to that?" "I guess you showed Germy who's the boss that time!" When you've finished the review, you can help the child sum up what you've all learned about OCD so far.

The most important message I can offer you at this point is to keep it light, brief, and casual. No arguments. You're establishing yourselves as part of a team working with your child to fight this intruder called OCD, and it all starts with kindness and trust.

Helping younger kids: For children under age 8 or so, or for any youngster who would rather draw than write, you may want to ask the child to review Step 1 in pictures rather than writing sentences. Other kids may just prefer to talk about how it works or doesn't work for them. Some kids will talk a lot; others very little. It doesn't matter so long as your child gets it. As you talk with your child, remember that winning at this stage is not getting rid of OCD but getting perspective on it—that is, not getting lost in OCD thoughts and rituals—and finding a common language to use that makes OCD like a third person in the room. That's it, and it is really important.

Helping teenagers: Teenagers, who typically call OCD by its medical name, generally find it helpful to become knowledgeable about the nature and causes of OCD. Most of this material can be found in Chapter 3, but the interested teen (and parents) may also want to look at some of the references at the back of this book. If your teenager has shown interest in learning more, can you help out by offering to find the material online or at the library? Your goal should be to know as much as or more than your doctors about OCD—I'm always pleased when one of my patients points out something I hadn't heard of before. Although this type of study may be helpful for younger kids, they typically do better talking than reading about it, because the material can get quite technical. The key point is that information is power.

Reviewing as a Family

OCD is irritating, no question about it. In fact, if it were fun, no one would want to work the program. More important, because the program works, your son or daughter, like others who've used it successfully, will want to keep at it for the simple reason that the child feels better. It's true that OCD will still be around at this point. In fact, it probably won't have changed all that much, but your child should still feel better. To test this out, you all might want to sit down to go over the following questions together informally and share your responses with each other.

1. How are we thinking about OCD differently? Is it clear to everyone that OCD is a medical illness like diabetes or asthma? Or does it still seem like something the child does on purpose?

2. What causes OCD? Does the fact that it's a brain hiccup make a difference in how we relate to it and to each other?

3. Are we parents (and your other kids) on the same page here? Does it seem like one person is too sympathetic and another judgmental and harsh? To make sure everyone is allied against OCD, can we come to see OCD as an illness that has little to do with good or bad behavior?

4. Can we tell what is OCD from what is not OCD? Are we more able to note the things that are OK rather than to focus only on problems related to OCD?

5. What does it mean to be patient and kind about OCD? How has doing this changed our willingness to work together to vanquish OCD? When we're impatient, what's the result? Do the rituals stop? Does our being impatient

make it easier to resist OCD, or is it just another obstacle to making progress?

6. How have we done in not giving unwanted advice about OCD? When advice is given, is it helpful?

7. Does everyone understand the program, especially how it unfolds over time? Are we all willing to sign on to the program, or is there still an "expert" in the crowd who wants to be in control? If so, what effect is this having on OCD?

Get Going

Make OCD the Problem

The only important tip for parents here is to help your child stick with the program. Use the chosen nickname or the term *OCD* to refer to OCD in the third person, remind yourself to talk about OCD as an impersonal illness, and encourage your child to do the same, using the questions listed in the kids' instructions as a template for practice.

Helping younger kids: Children under age 8 or so are too young to go through this practice completely on their own, so you may want to read these questions to younger kids. Keep it light and easy, a chance for the child to show his capability rather than a test that might conclude in some perception of failure. Although, as discussed in the preceding chapter, this program is not tied directly to any system of rewards, younger kids may respond well to receiving some small treat every time they sit through a short Q&A session with you.

Helping teenagers: Your teenager will probably want to answer these questions on her own, recording on paper any answers that surprise the teen or that she might not remember. Some teens find it worthwhile to keep a journal, but don't push that if yours doesn't want any more writing homework. The important thing is to get the idea and to practice it until it becomes second nature. As your teen learns to observe and to talk about OCD as a brain hiccup, she might want to review Chapter 3 to really instill the neurobiological basis of OCD. Then the teen can ask herself the questions, substituting "this illness," "this skipping CD," "this hiccup," or a similar phrase for "OCD."

How a therapist can help: Some parents may find it helpful to watch how a therapist poses these questions in an unthreatening, encouraging way that will motivate the child to do this preliminary work. The idea is to have the conversation go something like what you would expect if you visited a kind and compassionate specialist in the care of children with diabetes or asthma. You learn about the illness and what can be done to treat it so that you can get on with living your life as best you can. Then you go home and do what needs to be done to take good care of yourself.

Start to Map OCD

Making a map of OCD can provoke anxiety in many kids, at least at first, as they see how much OCD interferes in their lives. If your son or daughter is feeling dejected by OCD's large territory on the map, remind the child of all the positive elements in the child's life where OCD doesn't intrude. Accept with gentleness and compassion that OCD has a big hold on this child for the moment, while reminding him and yourself that this will change as you work through the program. Remember with deep respect the difficulty of resisting OCD and the achievements your child has already made since he started the program.

If your child shows signs of becoming anxious over the prospect of trying to boss back OCD in all the areas the child has already listed, gently point out how many of these triggers are high up on the fear thermometer and therefore won't be addressed at all for weeks ahead. She will choose how fast to go, and even then the rule is to stick to the work zone so that it will never be unmanageable. Except for the idea that everyone should always do the best he or she can in resisting OCD, everything above the work zone is off limits until, as the child goes up the ladder of difficulty, the harder tasks themselves come down (as they will) into the work zone.

If you can inject humor into your conversations about OCD, go ahead, but be sure you keep it gentle. This is not the place for sarcasm or overblown jokes. Think of it as aiming for gentle teasing of OCD rather than anything that might feel like mockery to your child.

> *I was making fun of OCD, doing parodies on Zach's nickname, even calling OCD Barney. Zach hates Barney (it's for little kids), and my making fun made him feel like I didn't understand how hard it was. Worse, he felt like I was making fun of him. Fortunately, I could see what was happening, so I asked him if I'd gone over the edge. We talked about it, which helped us both understand how OCD does and does not intrude into Zach's life.*
>
> —William, father of Zach (age 10)

Keep in mind that even using a nickname and poking fun at OCD is your child's very first sign of willingness to resist OCD, and for some children this can be a frightening step, especially if it gets OCD going. Remember what you know about your child, the unique individual who is not defined by OCD, and use that intimate knowledge to gauge when to hold back on gentle nudges forward versus poking fun at OCD.

> *One day, when we were joking about OCD, I said something I thought was innocuous about a really tough OCD symptom. Shana burst into tears and ran off to the bathroom, where she got stuck washing her hands for almost an hour. Just thinking about it got OCD rolling. Nothing I could say or do consoled her. When it was over—fortunately, because of the program I was sympathetic rather than*

mad—I told her I was sorry and we talked about how it had happened. It was really important to learn how much certain kinds of otherwise normal thoughts triggered OCD. Neither of us really appreciated this aspect of OCD before. After that, I was really careful not to overdo it.

—Alice, mother of Shana (age 8)

Helping younger kids: You'll have to help your child define the triggers for OCD symptoms. Use the map: trigger, obsession, compulsion. Sometimes there is no trigger. Lots of times there is no thought at all, just an urge or a feeling, such as the need to get something evened up, that defines the obsession. When there are only thoughts, try to tease apart the obsessions from the rituals. For example, if your child has bad thoughts that make him feel immoral or as if he's sinned, these are obsessions, whereas praying rituals to cancel out the obsessions are compulsions. As always, the key is to have a gentle, friendly, nonthreatening discussion about what OCD looks like and how it acts based on how you respond to it. Because talk about OCD and your child's behavior may very well have been unpleasant for all of you, you may have to approach this task gently and in stages to establish that you're completely uncritical. Be sure to acknowledge that now you see it differently, just as he does. Make suggestions to the child, saying things like "Sometimes OCD seems to get you particularly worried when . . ." and then wait for your child's affirmation, elaboration, or alternate explanation.

Parents will also have to present and explain drawings of the work zone to very young children. Instead of "work zone," consider developmentally appropriate terms from school, such as "science area" or something else your child will grasp.

Helping teenagers: Encourage your teenager to look ahead to Chapter 7 (pages 144–145) and review the Children's Yale–Brown Obsessive–Compulsive Scale symptom checklists to help him or her select the five to eight symptoms to begin mapping OCD. If the long list of symptoms seems like it might be overwhelming and too suggestive, offer to do this together.

How a therapist can help: If you're working with a therapist, she can help you refine the language you use to talk about OCD. Using the program, the therapist will model how to talk about OCD, so that this can become the pattern between you and your child and, more important, the pattern of conversation in your child as he talks to himself about OCD. Because most therapists are skilled at narrative interventions, she can guide you in this process, so that you become ever more subtle at identifying the ways in which OCD gets your child to confuse what it's doing with what he's doing. For example, there's a persistent invitation to refer to OCD as "your OCD" when OCD belongs to no one. It is completely impersonal, like hiccups or having to go to the bathroom. It just happens, and you have to respond. In conversation, the therapist, who's completely outside the circle, can identify these unwitting traps for you so you learn how not to fall into them. As always, if you're stuck and can't get unstuck, you'll need to find a therapist with expertise in the treatment of OCD.

Get to Know the Fear Thermometer

Here again, cheerleading from a place of understanding is your principal role. Where appropriate, try to clarify for yourself as much as for your child where OCD symptoms lie on the fear thermometer. Make sure you understand what's in the work zone, but don't encourage your child to resist more than she is doing already. Just doing the best she can is enough for now, as we don't want her to get beaten up by OCD for trying something too hard too soon. For many parents, identifying everything above the easy stuff is liberating, because knowing that these symptoms aren't approachable and so just have to be accepted for now makes it easier not to feel guilty or angry that you may not be doing enough. If you're having trouble with responding to OCD from a place of kindness and if this is making it hard to say things that help and don't hurt, try reading this poem from the Persian poet Rumi to each other. It may or may not help, but it's worth a good laugh and will remind you to relate to each other in a more helpful way.

"Relationship Booster"

Here is a relationship booster
that is guaranteed to
work.

Every time your friend says something stupid
make your eyes light up as if you

just heard something

brilliant.

It was so, so helpful to Luke and to us not to have to do anything other than accept that OCD is around for now. For Luke, the idea that he'd never have to do something that he wasn't already winning at some of the time took a lot of fear out of participating in the program. For me and his dad, knowing that we simply had to practice patience for the other stuff, even though OCD bugged us no end, made it much easier for us to agree on what to do. Not arguing about OCD all the time is really nice.

—Kathy, parent of Luke (age 11)

Jake and I used to fight all the time about what I called his "stupid quirks." Well, they are stupid, but now I know that it's OCD that's stupid and not Jake. After all these years, it's still hard for me not to be critical of him, but I'm getting better at it, and every time I do it I apologize. Yesterday, Jake told me not to apologize anymore as he understands that it's just a habit I'm trying to break. He asked me if I wanted to give it a nickname and set up a list. We both laughed. That made us feel much closer than we had in a long time.

—Doug, parent of Jake (age 17)

Helping younger kids: Instead of using the thermometer calibrated with numbers pictured in this chapter, consider drawing your own unlabeled thermometer and using a range of smiley to frowny faces. Then let your child color in the "mercury" to the point on the thermometer that represents how hard OCD is to resist.

Helping teenagers: Teenagers are likely to be very good at observing OCD symptoms, so they can jump the gun a bit and (1) use a 100-point scale to capture finer gradations in difficulty or (2) set up more than one checklist for different kinds of OCD, say one for contamination fears and rituals and another for religious obsessions and praying rituals. Ask your teenager if the fear thermometer in the kids' instructions seems too young and simplistic. If so, offer this alternative. Tell your teen to make sure when setting up the thermometer that he considers where the work zone is. Take a particular ritual (say washing) and try to place different ways to break OCD's rules on different parts of the hierarchy. For example, stopping washing altogether might be an 8, whereas getting one finger wrong out of the washing-fingers-in-a-certain-order required by OCD might be a 3. Getting pencils arranged just so at home might be a 3, but before a test at school might be a 7. Hearing the word "AIDS" might be a 3, looking at a picture of a person with AIDS in a magazine might be a 5, but touching someone with AIDS might be beyond a 10, for now anyway.

How a therapist can help: Some children who are afraid of OCD will "fake bad" or "fake good" so as to avoid having to confront OCD. This would mean a symptom list of all zeroes or all 10s, or sometimes kids will say "I can't think of anything." Here, too, a therapist skilled at drawing kids out can help garner accurate information and in so doing help a child master this task. When there is disagreement in the family about how something should be rated (easy versus hard), it is generally the person with OCD who knows best. If the disagreement leads to bad feelings, then you're stuck, and maybe a therapist can help you get unstuck.

Taking Stock

As at the end of Step 1, make sure your OCD scale and graph agree with your child's; if not, go back through this step and Step 1 to see where the disagreement arises. Also, as we said in the introduction to Part II, if your child doesn't find any of this record keeping helpful, junk the checklists and other forms, reserving them for your own use if you wish, but only if they are helpful to you. For kids who have organizational and writing problems, any writing homework is hard. Be a scribe when it's appropriate, or just use verbal stories to acknowledge what progress your child is making. Some people like to set up their own system for keeping track of progress on the computer, say, using Microsoft Outlook's planning function. Be creative, but do the program.

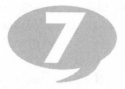

Step 3: Making a Map

A GOOD MAP will always help you get where you want to go. In your battle with OCD, the more you know about the territory you need to recover, the easier it is to triumph. You've done some preliminary scouting and know that you're stronger than you might have thought. In Step 3, you fill in the rest of your map so that you can begin to go after OCD where it's weakest.

The Game Plan for Step 3

A big part of Step 2 involved starting to make a map of OCD—what makes those OCD thoughts get started, what you do to try to make them go away or at least make yourself feel better while they're around, and how scary each usually is. Look at your list of five to eight symptoms now. Did you end up adding to it over the past week? Does it still seem right, or do you need to change any of the fear temperatures? How did you do in talking back to OCD?

Once you've done this quick review, follow the "Get Ready" directions. Then spend about a week following the instructions for this step. As before, do 30 to 60 minutes of work every day on everything you've learned through Step 3. You'll be adding in Step 4 before that time is up; 2 weeks for all of Steps 1–4 should be fine. At the end of this week, complete the OCD scale on page 95 again and add your ratings to the graph on page 96. Keep checking off the box for completing your homework each day on the "Getting Stronger Every Day" chart.

Here are a few tips for success during Step 3:

• Spend time wisely on the first steps. Sure, you need to feel comfortable that you're doing well with the tasks for each step before moving forward, but you don't want to be *too* cautious. Programs such as this one work because you build on your success: You see a change in how you're feeling, which naturally makes you want to keep going; you see another change, and you're raring to go on to the next step. Stay at one stage for too long and you feel stalled, as if you're just spinning the wheels on your bike—which makes you less eager to keep pedaling.

• *The map of OCD that you draw in Step 3 should be complete before you move on to Step 4.* Having a map with a lot of blank spaces would be like going into a football game without knowing where the end zone, goalposts, or 50-yard line is. You need that map before you start learning how to resist OCD at the next step.

• *Spend a lot of your daily homework time practicing the "brainpower" techniques in Goal 1 for this step.* These techniques will keep reminding you that OCD is a brain illness and help you label the symptoms as brain hiccups, things outside yourself that are impersonal and have no real meaning—fakes, despite the fact that they feel real. Talk kindly and realistically to yourself about the illness we call OCD and resolve to do something skillful about it. These tools are critical to helping you accomplish the tasks that you'll start trying out in Step 4.

Get Ready

Tear out the summary sheet for Step 3 from the back of this book or make a copy of it and stick it on your refrigerator, your bathroom mirror, your closet door, or wherever you're likely to see it most often. Talk to your parents about the map you started last week and see whether they have any ideas for revising or adding to it. Make sure your "Getting Stronger Every Day" chart is up-to-date—you're about to be able to start checking off the box for doing Step 3 homework.

Get Going

Brainpower: A New Way of Thinking about OCD

Boss Back OCD by Scouting It Out

During Steps 1 and 2, you started to shift the balance of power between you and OCD by talking back to OCD. You began to put OCD in its proper place by simply calling OCD by its own name or giving it a funny nickname. You went on to learn that OCD is an illness that most kids can recover from, a hiccup in one small part of the brain, and if you didn't know it before, you know now that you're not crazy, weird, or doomed to insanity. You don't do these things; OCD does. Or, rather, OCD makes you do them, and you just need to learn how to be the boss of OCD instead of the other way around. Saying "I'm the boss" in situations that don't feel too scary and then noticing that OCD hasn't made you feel even worse should be giving you the idea that OCD isn't so big and tough after all—at least not everywhere, all the time. You may have tried challenging OCD's threats, telling OCD things like "I don't have to count every step I take while I'm at school" or "Nothing bad will happen to my family just because OCD put these nasty ideas in my head." If doing so made you too frightened to go on or even made you feel like you had to perform one of your rituals right then and there, step back a little and try a more general type of talking back: "Look, I may have had to do the ritual this time, but just knowing that this is OCD and not me is progress." The more you talk back to OCD, the more you get a feel for when and where you can win without much effort and where it's much harder. Keep it up over the next week, noticing which situations get easier and which ones stay hard. Pay particular attention to how talking back to OCD works with the symptoms (hiccups) you listed in Step 2. If you can, jot down some notes about how you feel and what you do when you talk back to OCD in different settings.

Give Yourself a Pep Talk

Most kids and teenagers with OCD find themselves stuck in a painful spot: They feel they have no power against OCD, yet they put themselves down for performing rituals, especially when the rituals interfere with schoolwork or home life. Blaming yourself is one reason you've probably noticed that you feel worse before, during, and after rituals now than you did in the past. Also, blaming yourself makes it harder to get the most you can out of the strategies you'll learn starting in Step 4.

An important kind of brainpower here is to give yourself a break. When you feel like you have to wash your hands or check a lock or make sure you've saved all the wrappers from the little toys you get at the local fast-food place, don't beat yourself up over it. Don't agonize over whether you're letting OCD win again or whether the rituals will get worse (as they probably have over time). Instead of saying to yourself "What if I have to wash my hands for even longer this time?" try thinking "I'm just going to do the best I can to do as little OCD as possible." If that kind of statement ends up making you feel really frightened or upset, try just saying "It's OK if I can't stop doing these rituals right now. I'm building my toolkit, and soon I'll be able to start resisting OCD." Giving yourself a break will serve you well until the very end of this book, when you'll get to the most difficult items on your list of OCD symptoms.

Cut OCD Down to Size

You already know OCD has a bad deal to offer: Perform this ritual, says OCD, and whatever you're afraid will happen won't come true. Refuse to perform the ritual, and your worst fears *will* come true. I hope you're beginning to believe that OCD doesn't deserve your trust. OCD says it's 100% certain that if you touch a plant and then your mother without washing your hands, you'll pass on germs to her that will make her sick. Or that if you don't check 20 times to make sure the door is locked, criminals will break into your house, and your family will be hurt. When you get confused and think OCD is telling the truth, you feel like you have to do what OCD says.

To avoid this, let's look at what OCD has to say using our own brainpower rather than relying on OCD to tell the truth. Though this sort of approach applies most to OCD symptoms that involve harm, it is definitely a better way to argue with OCD. Pretend you're a newspaper reporter and investigate whether OCD is telling the truth by asking three questions: What is the chance something bad will happen? How bad will it be? Am I really responsible?

• *What is the chance that what OCD says will happen*? How often has your mother gotten sick recently? Maybe she had a cold last winter or a stomach virus last month, but she's probably not always sick, is she? Yet she touches the plants every day when she waters them. So, OCD may say there's a 100% chance of your mother getting sick if you touch a plant and then her without washing your hands, but if you think about it, what's the realistic chance? Zip, really! And what if your mother does get sick from time to time? How likely is it that OCD is right about what caused her to get sick? Pretty silly, right? OCD says that germs on a plant caused it, but you know better. So tell yourself that you're smarter than OCD— because you are. When OCD tries to convince you otherwise, don't doubt yourself; just label OCD as OCD and move on.

• *How bad will it be*? OCD says your mom won't just get sick; she'll get really sick, maybe even die. Sometimes people do get very sick, but usually OCD tells you always to fear the worst. You can remind yourself that getting sick is common, getting really sick isn't common, and dying doesn't happen very often and never because OCD says so. Put simply, you can say to OCD, "You worry too much."

• *Am I really responsible*? OCD plays a particularly cruel trick by trying to get you to blame yourself if something happens. That way you'll be even more likely to do rituals. So ask yourself the following question: "If Mom gets sick, how likely is it that I'm the one who's responsible for passing those germs on?" Make a pie chart like the one below. Tell yourself, "Maybe she got the flu at work or from a friend, or from who-knows-where, but it definitely isn't because of me."

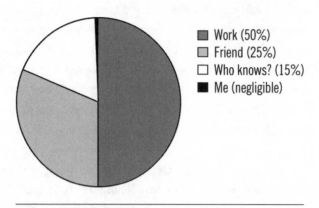

Pie chart you can use to check whether OCD is telling the truth (in this case, about where your mother might catch an illness).

So even though you're probably not ready to resist washing your hands every time you touch a plant, you can think different thoughts when OCD tells you there's a 100% chance that if you don't wash your hands after touching a plant, your mother will get sick. You can say, "It's not too likely that Mom will get sick, and if she does it's not too likely that it came from the plant, and it certainly won't be my fault. Sorry, OCD, but I'm not buying it. What you say is not what I say!"

Let OCD Float By

This is probably the most important brainpower tool of all. Every time you call OCD by its name or the nickname you've given it, you disown it, telling OCD you know it's separate from you. It's not you who came up with obsessions and compulsions; it's the illness we call OCD. Now we're going to ask you to use your brainpower to step back from OCD even further. If you think about OCD for a minute, it will be obvious that OCD comes and goes in its own time, the same way the wind blows, the rain falls, birds fly above you, and the clouds float through the sky. OCD arises sometimes in response to triggers and at other times just on its own, but you don't do anything to make it happen. It just happens; it also goes away on its own. You think that doing rituals makes OCD let go, but scientific studies have shown that if you didn't do the rituals, OCD would hang around for just about the same amount of time. Do the rituals and it's there for 45 minutes; don't do the rituals—

still there for 45 minutes. At least this is probably your experience at this point. As you'll see when you start working your way through this program, when you put into action a plan for *not* doing the rituals and stick with that plan time after time when OCD comes up, OCD will stop showing up.

Now try *not* to think about something—for example, a pink elephant. What happened? You thought about it more, right? More and more scientific studies tell us that trying to block something from your mind just makes it pop up even stronger. Sometimes jerking your mind away from OCD or even arguing with it is the most skillful thing you can do. Sometimes not: OCD can get worse when you try to suppress it, and when this happens the best thing to do is just to look at it as though it's like a bit of bad weather passing through. Remind yourself that OCD is as meaningless as a hiccup. These are not your thoughts, and they are no more real than what happens on TV. They're just passing phenomena that you can watch knowing that they don't in any way belong to your sense of who you are. Whatever you do, don't identify OCD with yourself. Treat OCD just like a cloud in the sky: You see it, you recognize it for what it is, you label it unimportant, and you go about your business. It isn't real, so why push it away? Getting all wound up about obsessions and performing rituals are what keeps OCD in charge. Shed the struggle and don't do rituals, and OCD eventually moves on, just like cloudy weather. If you have the doubting form of OCD, and OCD is forever trying to get you to figure out whether something is OCD or not, this brainpower tool is particularly useful. Just label "figuring it out" as doubting, know that it is OCD, and don't get lost in a mental hurricane of thinking about it. Instead, relax, accept that OCD is present, and move on to something else, while waiting for OCD to get bored and go away on its own. Remember, the essence of brainpower is to observe OCD at a distance so you are never lost in it—just see clearly whatever flavor of OCD is arising, label it as OCD, and respond as skillfully as you can in that moment. There's nothing more you can do, and if you master the program, this will be enough in the end.

Making statements like the ones in the box on the next page doesn't mean you avoid OCD triggers or obey OCD and perform rituals and *then* laugh it off, as if it doesn't matter. Being sick has real meaning and requires that you and your family respond skillfully. OCD just isn't a very good playmate. If you ignore it, it'll soon get bored and leave you alone. If you argue, let it in, and then struggle a lot, OCD wins and will keep bugging you, so try to remember to let OCD go.

Which Kind of Brainpower to Use When?

Sometimes one or another of the brainpower techniques just described will be easier to use than in others. Or you'll find that one works better in some situations

When OCD makes an appearance, try saying the following things (or something like them) to yourself:

1. "Oh, it's just OCD again." To avoid getting upset, some kids find it helpful to add nonchalantly, "Hi, OCD [or Germy, or Dodohead, or whatever nickname you've chosen]. Don't have time to play with you today."
2. "My brain is just hiccupping again." You know OCD appears because electric circuits in your brain are misfiring, and this is a way to remind yourself at a time when OCD is likely to try other guises.
3. "These hiccups aren't important, because they aren't real." You don't need to do anything except just patiently wait OCD out, because what OCD says is meaningless.
4. "I guess I'll just do something I like until OCD goes away." You don't need to take any directions from OCD, so you might as well have some fun until OCD gets bored with your ignoring it. Hey, congratulations! You just did something in response to OCD besides doing rituals!

than in others. Or one will work best at a specific time in a run-in with OCD but not so well at other times (such as when OCD shows up when you've already started to try to resist it). Always feel free to use all the techniques in whatever combination is easiest and works best for you.

It's really hard for me to get into school if the door's not propped open. If I see it closed, Grimy starts right in with "Oh, no, it's so dirty. Just think of how many kids touched that handle! Where do you think they put their hands before they came to school?!" If I have time before school, what works best for me is to pull out my pie chart and remind myself that my new baby brother isn't gonna get sick just because I touched the school door, and babies get over being sick real fast anyway. It's no big deal. But if I'm in a big hurry that day, I try giving myself a pep talk on the bus: "Grimy's not gonna get to me today, because I am on top of this!" But if Grimy still pops up real loud when I get to school, I just stop halfway down the front walk and pull out my little photo album where I keep pictures of my new puppy (yeah, we got him pretty much at the same time as we got my brother!). He's so cute I just start laughing, and I look at the pictures till Grimy drifts away, which really only takes about 3 minutes these days. I don't even miss the first bell anymore.

—Sasha, age 12

Like Sasha, you will probably find out quickly that your brainpower tools work best for you in a certain order. Or you may just know from reading about the techniques which ones you'd want to try first when OCD comes up. Some kids find it helpful to write down their responses to OCD on an index card that they can carry with them. You can do this in whatever way works best for you. Sasha might write down her brainpower tools as reminders to herself, in which case her first one might be "1. Remember, OCD makes no sense!" Or she might write her own lines, as if they are part of a script she needs to practice whenever OCD comes up: "2. No way are you gonna win today, OCD, because I *rule.*" Having this brainpower card with you can really help you focus on using your tools when OCD interrupts your day and you feel that you're too upset to know what to do.

For teenagers: You may be at the point in your life when you don't particularly like doing anything that your parents tell you to—even if it's what you want to do anyway. If you find yourself resisting your parents instead of concentrating on learning to resist OCD, try suggesting—gently, if you possibly can—that when your parents feel anxious about whether you're doing your part to eliminate OCD, or when they seem to be interfering too much, they simply ask, "What can I do to be helpful?" and leave it at that. There may be times when you want your parents intimately involved and other times when you do not. So long as the program is going well, you're fine either way.

How a therapist can help: Doing the program is easy if you can get unstuck when things don't go so well. If you feel like you're stuck trying to get the brainpower skills to work, or if you just can't get into the habit of using them, a therapist can help. Also, if you feel that OCD gets worse whenever you try talking back to it, you may be trying to do too much too soon. But instead of just slowing down, talk to your therapist. As we mentioned earlier in this chapter, slowing down too much can get you stalled; a therapist can help you figure out whether you're having problems because you're speeding or because something else is tripping you up.

Complete Your Map of OCD

You started mapping OCD during Step 2, when you listed five to eight symptoms in your chart, including the trigger (if any), the obsession, the compulsion, and how much fear OCD made you feel. You learned about the work zone, the area in which you're already successful at resisting OCD more than half of the time. The work zone includes all the territory not clearly owned by either you or OCD. By working on the OCD symptoms from the work zone during later steps, you'll start chipping away at OCD's territory so that yours grows and grows. One reason this program is so successful is that we take something you're already partially successful at and convert it into 100% success. Everything outside the work zone is off limits, except that you do the best you can. To be sure you know what to do and what you shouldn't tackle yet, you need a complete map of OCD. This is your next task, and it's important, so take your time and be sure to stick with it until you feel confident that your map (your chart of symptoms) is done.

Start by looking at the chart with your five to eight symptoms. Do you want to change anything now that you've been watching OCD pull its tricks over the last several days? Is the temperature rating still accurate? If not, make whatever changes you need to make. The boy whose sample "map" you saw on page 125 made a few changes: OCD hadn't been giving him much trouble over the dog, so he changed the fear temperature for petting the dog to a 3 instead of a 3-4. He'd gotten his hair cut short, though, and ever since then, OCD had been making him comb his hair over and over till it felt right on both sides of his head; he added that hiccup to his chart and assigned it a 5 on the fear thermometer. He also added a "just so" obsession that had to do with getting his covers tucked in just right when he went to bed and having the curtains closed so that they met nice and evenly.

Now you're going to add to your list. To help kids draw a complete map, therapists use a couple of checklists. These checklists were written based on talks with lots of kids who are struggling with OCD, just as you are. The obsessions and compulsions that bug you may not be just like any one other boy or girl's, but OCD isn't really a very original thinker, and so we see a lot of the same types of symptoms over and over again. Lots of kids have the same obsessions and the same rituals, so don't be ashamed to check off whatever symptoms apply to you.

The most common obsessions and compulsions are listed here. If you want a more detailed list, the original therapist's checklist is on page 266 at the back of the book. Take an hour or so of time when you're feeling relaxed and won't have to rush off to do homework or get to baseball practice and check off the OCD symptoms that affect you as honestly as you can. Don't get stuck and don't think too hard. At first, just quickly check off the symptoms that are part of OCD's bag of tricks.

Common OCD Symptoms

Obsessions:

- ☐ Upset about dirt, germs, chemicals, radiation, or sticky things
- ☐ Responsible for bad things happening
- ☐ May cause someone to get sick or hurt
- ☐ Bad or silly thoughts about getting sick
- ☐ May cause myself or someone else to get sick or hurt
- ☐ Get worried about sin or wrongdoing for no reason

☐ Have bad thoughts about sex

☐ Trouble making my mind up (doubting)

☐ Other bad/silly thoughts that I can't stop (name)

Compulsions:

☐ Reread/rewrite for no reason

☐ Have to wash or clean for no reason

☐ Check that nothing bad happened

☐ Check things over and over again for no reason

☐ Keep things straight, even, or balanced

☐ Can't throw things away

☐ Count things for no reason

☐ Have to figure things out (doubting)

☐ Have to move or talk in a special way

☐ Have to say prayers, ask for reassurance, or apologize for no reason

☐ Repeat things for no reason

☐ Do things over and over until it feels just right

☐ Touch things for no reason

☐ Pick skin, bite nails, pull hair

☐ Think some part of my body is really ugly

☐ Other things I have to do over and over for no reason (name)

Once you've checked off the OCD symptoms that you think you currently have, see if you can put each OCD symptom into your own words. Be as specific as you can. For example, if you checked off germ worries and washing rituals, you'd write something along the lines of "I'll get germs on my hands and something bad will happen to my mom, so I have to wash my hands five times after touching the sink or toilet." If you checked off causing something bad to happen and checking, you might write "I have to check to be sure my bad thoughts didn't cause my dad to be in a bad accident."

Now enter obsessions in the "Obsession" column of your chart, with the compulsions in the "Compulsions" column. You may have one or more than one ritual for each obsession; just list them all in as much detail as you can. Don't forget to enter things OCD makes you avoid, such as touching the bathroom sink or toilet, as a compulsion, too.

Now think about what triggers each obsession and compulsion. If you're worried that something bad will happen to anyone you touch because you have germs on your hand, the trigger might be touching the bathroom sink or touching the toilet—or both. If more than one thing triggers a particular obsession, enter all the triggers separately and just repeat the obsession (or use "ditto" marks). As suggested in Step 2, if you want you can divide up your list into sublists by "flavor" of OCD: washing, checking, ordering or arranging, counting or repeating, moral or religious OCD, and hoarding.

Now use the fear thermometer that you added to your toolkit in Step 2 to figure out the fear temperature of each entry in your chart and enter it as shown on the completed chart on the next page.

Over the next week, your job is to see how complete this list is. You're still a detective. You might want to keep a little notebook for taking informal notes about your encounters with OCD over the next several days:

- How does OCD arise? Does it just show up in your mind as a mental hiccup? Are there triggers for OCD that you can avoid? Triggers that you can avoid or can only avoid with real difficulty?
- See where you beat OCD all of the time, some of the time, and hardly ever. Do you ever choose to confront an OCD trigger? Refrain from doing rituals? You'll use this information to see how accurate the fear temperatures you've entered are and to make changes as necessary.
- Pay attention to how much time is spent on each obsession. How many minutes or hours a day would you say you spend on each one? Or, if these thoughts pop into your head quickly and then leave, how often do they come up? Jot down times for each day over the next week. How much time do you spend on compulsions? Jot this down, too.
- How much do obsessions interfere with your life at home, at school, and with your friends? How about compulsions?
- How much do obsessions bother you? How upset do you get over compulsions?
- How hard do you try to resist obsessions? What about compulsions? (Don't take this question as nagging. As we said earlier in Step 3, you can try bossing back OCD a little, but don't push it yet.)
- How often can you control obsessions? Is it easier if you just let OCD float by and go on about your business?
- What people, places, or things do you avoid because of obsessions or so you won't feel that you have to perform a ritual?

Many kids use a little scale—like the one on the fear thermometer but shorter—to record their answers to these questions: 1 for mild, 2 for moderate, 3 for severe, and 4 for extreme. If that's helpful to you, you can use it. At first, though, many kids just like to take notes.

Action/situation/trigger	Obsession	Compulsion	Temp. (1–10)
WASHING			
Touching toilet	"I'll get germy and make Mom sick."	Avoid touching toilet or wash hands 5 times.	10
Using friend's bathroom	"I'll get their family's germs and make my family sick."	Avoid visiting for long enough to need the bathroom.	8
Touching my mouth with my fingers	"I'll get sick and die from germs on my hands."	Wash hands every time my fingers touch my mouth.	6
Touching doorknobs	"I'll get people's germs and get sick."	Use shirt, tissue, or coat to hold doorknobs.	6
Petting the dog	"The dog's germs will spread and make everyone sick."	Pet dog with gloves on or wash hands 5 times.	3
Walking by dog after shower	Ditto	Don't walk within 6 feet of the dog.	1–2
ORDERING OR ARRANGING			
Getting dressed for school	"I have to make sure my socks are evened up."	Even up socks over and over until they feel right. Ask Mom whether they look straight.	5
Ditto	"I have to make sure my hair is combed evenly."	Comb hair over and over until it looks right in the mirror.	5
Going to bed	"The curtains need to be closed evenly so they meet right in the center of the window."	Pull curtains closed, step back to check them, then adjust them over and over.	3–4
Ditto	"My covers have to be folded over evenly when Mom tucks me in."	Mom has to keep tucking them in until they feel right to me.	3
Getting dressed for school	"My watch has to be right in the middle of my wrist."	Don't wear watch or adjust it on my wrist till it looks right.	1–2

Over the next week, use the information you jot down to revise your chart if you get the idea that a trigger is not as big a deal as you thought or if you've left one out altogether, and so forth.

While you're recording information about OCD's impact on your life, don't forget one very important thing: When and where are you free of OCD's grip during the day? Where can you go to have fun even when OCD is hanging around? If you jot down those places where OCD has a hard time getting you lost in the illness, you'll get a lot of information about your strengths, and as we go along you can build on those. Pay particular attention to what you enjoy doing and where you feel brave and are willing to take risks (such as on the soccer field or during a math test).

For teenagers: You might want to ask for your parents' review of your map in case you've left anything out. This is especially important if your parents or siblings are also tangled up in OCD symptoms. It can also help them understand how OCD works and, most important, get them off your back about OCD symptoms that are too high on the fear thermometer chart to tackle at the moment.

How a therapist can help: Some kids are so embarrassed about or ashamed of some of the obsessive thoughts that OCD puts in their head that they find it hard to talk about them and even hard to list them on their maps. It's really important not to let shame stand in the way of your making an accurate map of OCD. Can you remind yourself that OCD is sending you junk mail, spamming you, just like what happens on your computer? These things aren't personal—you don't own them; they just happen. If that doesn't help, you might need a kick start to make a map. A therapist will know how to talk with you so you don't feel personally responsible for OCD's ideas and so you know what belongs on your map and in your notes.

Reward Yourself for Progress Made

You're probably pretty used to beating yourself up over "giving in" to OCD. You may even feel like you're letting down your mom and dad or your brothers and sisters or your teachers and friends. Maybe you've gotten the idea that they think you should just be able to "control yourself" and that they don't understand that right now it's OCD that's in control. One of the main purposes for doing all this mapping work is to help you see what you're doing right. Besides reminding yourself of all the good parts of your life, we want you to get rewarded for any way that you're able to resist OCD. Here are some possibilities:

- Every time you catch yourself successfully bossing back OCD, congratulate yourself with a silent (or at least quiet—you don't want to disrupt your class or interrupt the TV show your family is watching) "Way to go!" or "I'm a genius!" or "I'm getting tougher every day!" You get the idea—your own words will be better than ours.

- Record the times you boss back OCD, either with a little note or by keeping a chart where you add a star for each time you beat OCD. This will help you locate the work zone. If you want, you can bring your record to your parents at the end of each day so they can reward you.
- Ask your parents to come up with a system of rewards you can earn for resisting OCD—and be sure to have them include some surprises.

For teenagers: Put simply, knowing that you're facing OCD rather than running from it is the only reward that really matters. Still, it's nice to have hard work recognized. You can probably reward yourself, the way adults often do when they're trying to motivate themselves to stick with something difficult, like dieting or quitting smoking. For example, you might get yourself a new CD. Or you might find longer-term, cumulative rewards more appealing. Ask your parents to come up with a modest amount of money (or something else) that they can add to a "bank" for you and then turn over the proceeds to you at the end of the week. Or designate a larger prize or privilege you want to work toward: earning the money for a videogame, a trip, or some new camping gear.

Taking Stock

Turn to the OCD scale again and complete it one more time. Add these scores to the graph you started making at the end of Step 1. Are you seeing any progress? It may be small, but it will definitely represent a downward trend for OCD—and an upward trend for you. Keep up the great work!

Have you been filling in your "Getting Stronger Every Day" chart? Before you move on to Step 4, you should feel like you're beginning to call in the brainpower techniques a little more automatically when OCD rears its head. You should feel confident that your map of OCD is complete and that you're taking regular notes about all the symptoms you've included in it so that your picture of OCD is getting clearer and clearer. And, finally, you should be starting to pat yourself on the back, mentally and through some kind of real rewards, for making headway against OCD by using all these strategies so far. If this describes how you feel and what you've accomplished, you're ready to add the Step 4 tasks to your regular homework. If not, give yourself another day or so, as long as you haven't gone beyond the 2-week mark. If 2 weeks have already passed and you don't feel at all ready for Step 4—if OCD is just too tough—talk to your parents about whether you need a therapist to help you.

Step 3: Instructions for Parents

The Game Plan for Step 3

Here's how you can help promote your child's progress:

• *Spend time wisely on the first steps.* Slow and steady may win the race in most cases, but for our purposes steady is more important than slow. It's especially important to complete the first four steps inside of 2 weeks so that kids can get to the steps that will let them see OCD symptoms start to be eliminated left and right. If your child is having trouble with any particular step, especially at these early stages, talk to a therapist right away.

• *The map of OCD that your child draws in Step 3 should be reasonably complete before the child moves on to Step 4.* Your input should be supportive instead of critical, but here's where you should make sure your child has accomplished what the step is designed to do. If your child has omitted OCD symptoms that you notice regularly, gently nudge him to think about whether something else is missing and offer hints to head him in the direction of adding these symptoms to his map. For children with "hidden" obsessions—where even talking about them is talking back to OCD— encourage the child to put them on the map even though that's hard to do in and of itself. He can always label the symptom or trigger as OCD X and use naming it as a task to be accomplished. When, starting in Step 4, your child assigns himself exposure tasks, one of these tasks will be expressing these obsessions out loud. For now, let the child know that it's fine not to say anything specific yet. Just reinforce the fact that these OCD thoughts are not real, not his, and that it's important to tell himself that these are not his thoughts and that he simply needs to label them as OCD.

• *Your child should spend a good portion of the daily homework time practicing the "brainpower" techniques in Goal 1 for this step.* This is another area in which you can be of help to your child, through gentle questions that encourage your child to build these skills (see the box on page 153).

Get Going

Brainpower: A New Way of Thinking about OCD

Parents always need to know the answer to a simple question: Is it *can't* or is it *won't*? OCD is mostly a *can't* problem, unlike refusing to clean one's room, which is a *won't*. The trick, which we'll help you with, is to tell them apart. If you play a significant role in your child's OCD, such as running the dishwasher three times so the dishes are "really clean" or letting your child stay up late to make sure all the windows and doors are locked before going to bed, you may need to learn to talk back to OCD, too. When you try to help your child by participating in rituals, you too are being bossed around by OCD, and you don't have to be. We'll help you get disentangled from OCD as we go along.

In the meantime, assume that OCD is always a *can't* and try to do what you can to be helpful. For example, you might remind your child that even though it doesn't feel good to get nervous or upset about an obsession or a compulsion, she can get through it just resisting OCD as well as she can at this point. "Do the best you can" is the maxim. After all, you're just getting started building the toolkit. Be sure not to push it too hard. Make yourself intimately familiar with the fear temperatures of various triggers on your child's growing map and be especially positive and encouraging when your child is trying to resist an OCD symptom that has a very low fear temperature. Everything else is off limits as too hard to encourage resistance. Remember that doing rituals at this point is OK, as everyone is doing the best he or she can, including you.

During this week, your child will find some of the brainpower techniques easier to use than others, or more effective in some situations than others, or effective at different points in an encounter with OCD. Most kids will end up blending all the brainpower tools when OCD shows up, in whatever combination they find easiest and most successful. You can help tremendously here, noting which tools seem to assuage your child's fear most quickly, which are easiest to use, or what order seems to work best. Once your child starts trying formal exposure and response prevention tasks, she will need to have a plan for use of these tools, so the greater extent to which you can figure out what sequence works best now, the farther ahead of the game you will be.

Use of these brainpower tools has to take into account your child's maturity and abilities, and you probably know those better than anyone else. You'll know when a technique is over your child's head and can help adapt it to the child's developmental age. It's also important to match the tool with the kind of OCD symptoms that bother your child.

Alex is a 6-year-old with tapping rituals. OCD makes Alex tap two times on his left and then two times on his right whenever he goes through a door. If he touches one leg or one ear, he has to tap the other one, both twice. Sometimes he isn't sure, so he has to start over. Because Alex knows that 2 × 2 is 4, OCD often makes him tap four times. Sometimes he has to start over if someone in the family interrupts him, which they are likely to do if he's blocking the door. This makes him mad. Alex taps because he has the urge to do so, and this urge also insists that things be even or balanced. There are no thoughts and definitely no fear of harm. He just feels that he has to do it and gets very uncomfortable if he doesn't, so he does it to get it over with hundreds of time each day. The tools that helped him get over OCD included naming it, understanding that his brain had the hiccups, and letting the urge come and go without struggling while doing something else more fun. Worries about consequences and responsibility don't apply, so his mom didn't teach him this tool. Everyone got with the program and made sure not to interrupt Alex during a ritual so that he didn't have to start over, thereby helping Alex instead of OCD.

Letting OCD float by like a burst of bad weather is a very good tool, but it's important for you and your child to understand that using this tool doesn't mean that your child avoids OCD triggers or performs rituals and *then* laughs it off. The point of letting OCD float by is that OCD depends on getting a reaction; when your child just lets OCD come and go without reacting to it, it tends to dissipate naturally. That's easier said than done, of course, and takes a lot of practice. If you like this tool, Jeff Schwartz, MD, in his wonderful book *Brain Lock*, talks a lot about it, and Jeff Brantley, in his book *Calming Your Anxious Mind*, on applying mindfulness to anxiety, does the same (see the Resources at the back of this book).

Helping younger kids: Younger kids may have a bit harder time internalizing a lot of these brainpower techniques. When practicing, they may benefit from talking back to OCD out loud, at least at first. When you hear the language the child uses in talking back, detaching a bit from OCD, or giving himself a pep talk, you'll know whether it is helpful at all and how well it works. Does your child seem calmer, happier, and better able to resist doing rituals? If not, help your child come up with age-appropriate words that he or she will remember and that will be understandable and relevant. Humor or levity may help some kids relax and let go of anxiety quickly. Encouraging your child to say "Uh-uh-uh, OCD, you're not as tricky as you think," while wagging his finger at OCD, might strike your child as funny and therefore release tension. Other kids may find acting like the hero or soldier more empowering and thus comforting: "Take that, OCD, you weakling" may work for some, but you'll need to make sure that the child's approach is not too belligerent or threatening, which may backfire.

When you're helping your child realistically assess the risks that OCD says she's taking if she doesn't obediently perform OCD's rituals, keep in mind that younger

---

Prompts You Can Use to Help Your Child Use the Brainpower Techniques

"Is OCD trying to get you to believe his nasty ideas again?"

"Is it getting a little easier to talk back to OCD at times like this?"

"Is it still hard to talk back to OCD in these places?"

"How do you feel when you talk back to OCD here?"

When the child feels ashamed of not being able to resist OCD:

"Did you remember that you're doing the best you can and you're sticking with it?"

"Even when OCD gets going, just note that it is present, relax as best you can, and try to do the most skillful thing in response to OCD that you know you can do."

"Maybe you couldn't resist OCD this time, but don't you think OCD knows you're not buying his story anymore?"

To remind the child to let OCD float by:

"Gee, I guess OCD just blew through again."

"Should we play cards for a few minutes till OCD gets bored hanging around here?"

"How are you doing on that new computer game? Feel like taking another shot at it?"

"Tell me about the game today—I heard you scored a goal!"

---

children often find the whole concept of probability and percentages very difficult to understand. If you see your child's eyes glaze over when you ask her to tell you what the chance is that her fears will be realized, you can skip this technique altogether. Instead, focus on convincing your child that she can't possibly be responsible for your illnesses, for the whole family's safety, for the salvation of anyone's soul, or for anything other than the tasks you've assigned her that suit her age, like making her bed, doing her homework, and being polite to adults.

If you think there's a chance that estimation of risk might be understandable to your child, the key is to connect your statements to the child's direct experience. It's hard for some kids to state what the realistic likelihood is that their mothers will get sick, but they may grasp what you're getting at if you ask them how often they've seen their mothers get sick—during this school year, or last year, or the year before that. Whatever you do, stick to the tools. That's especially true if you've been sick.

Even if you have been ill or if something has happened that is conceptually linked to OCD, that doesn't make OCD any less nonsensical. The idea here is not to give advice that OCD is silly and that the child should just stop. The idea here is to learn a specific tool to use during exposure and response prevention (EX/RP) tasks so that the probability of completing an EX/RP task successfully is increased. Don't expect your child to stop doing all rituals; do expect her to learn and practice the tool.

Helping teenagers: Most teenagers work better on their own than when their parents are hovering over them—and even if they don't, they prefer to do it that way. As in Step 2, you might encourage your teen to keep a journal of whatever depth he's comfortable with, recording successes or problems with the various brainpower techniques, with the goal of coming up with his own program for ongoing use. Depending on whether your teen and you have had a long history of fighting over OCD, you may have a hard time staying out of it. You may forget that no one hates OCD more than your teenager does. Remind yourself that, given half a chance, your teenager will do whatever he has to do to get rid of OCD. Remember that your son would much rather do what he needs to do because he wants to than because you are "making" him do it. When you're worried about whether your daughter is doing what she should to fight OCD, simply ask, "What can I do to be helpful?" and leave it at that. So, if you find your teen resisting you instead of concentrating on learning to resist OCD, try suggesting—gently, if you possibly can—that there may be times when she wants her parents intimately involved and other times when she does not. So long as the program is going well, you're fine either way.

How a therapist can help: Sometimes you and your child are so tangled up by OCD, by other disruptive behaviors (like ADHD), or by some combination of the two that your relationship just isn't enough to make this part of the toolkit work. Or maybe OCD is just too hard, or your child has given up and doesn't have the motivation to go on with the program. If this is the case—and it is pretty common for it to be this way—don't give up. Just find a trained CBT therapist and use the program under the therapist's guidance, folding in other interventions, such as parent training for ADHD, that may be helpful as well (see Resources).

Complete the Map of OCD

The only way to be certain about what your child can and should be doing to try to fight OCD and what's not possible for the time being is to be absolutely sure your child has a complete and accurate map. Don't nag your child over this. If there's one thing your child doesn't need while doing the hard but essential work of mapping OCD, it's helpful criticism. But do insist that this part of the program get the attention it deserves. Help him refine his map, asking your child to tell you about the fear temperature of triggers encountered and encouraging him to be a sharp detective in identifying triggers and difficult situations so that the OCD map can be completed accurately. Ask to see the map and encourage your child to talk about whether she feels it's complete and why. What can she tell you about how she's been observing

OCD over the past week or so to see what kinds of obsessions and compulsions OCD forces on her?

The checklists in the kids' section of Step 3 are included in one of the rating scales we first mentioned in Chapter 2, specifically, the Children's Yale–Brown Obsessive Compulsive Scale (CY-BOCS). You may want to familiarize yourself with this scale, which is included on pages 266–269 at the back of the book, to see whether any symptom not included on the simplified lists within the chapter is a part of your child's OCD. You can help your child fill out his map of OCD by identifying triggers that he has overlooked, but be gentle and very matter-of-fact when talking about obsessions and compulsions. Don't assume that you know everything there is to know about OCD—by now I'm never surprised to discover that the child has been wrestling with some sort of OCD that no one else knows about.

If your child has kept notes, praise her for doing so and offer to review them with her at the end of each day. But if all the record keeping seems overwhelming to your child, offer to be the "secretary" for the week—at least some of the time. Remember, too, that kids already have a lot of homework, and if your child doesn't want to write or has trouble with writing, skip the journaling and focus on doing the program.

If your child forgets to notice where OCD doesn't interfere in his life or what his positive traits are, remind him. Help your child think about where and how she wins over OCD: "Since OCD forced its way in here, how did you manage to keep it out of [name another area where the child beats OCD]?" This not only reminds the child that she can win but also helps her start thinking about what works well for her in resisting OCD without your insisting that she try harder to do so.

Helping younger kids: Much of the map making may be up to you if your child is young enough to be a new reader. Tell your child that you're going to draw a map so that the child can run OCD off his land. Initiate a dialogue that is gently probing: "Let's talk about the 'silly worries' that keep bothering you. . . . What happens when you need to use the bathroom? . . . I've heard that OCD sometimes makes other kids feel like they have to wash their hands in a certain way. Let's write down the way OCD tells you to do it." With very young children, whose insight may not be as sharp and whose powers of observation and reporting are immature, you will have to be more active in filling out the symptom list yourself.

Helping teenagers: Adolescents should be able to complete their maps pretty

---

Wording is important when you're helping your child map OCD.

Instead of "You always get upset when we don't clean the table settings right before we sit down to eat."

Say "OCD gets really bossy at dinnertime and wants us to clean the plates before we sit down."

much on their own, but if the teen wants to involve you, so much the better. If you or your other kids are tangled up in OCD, it might help your teen for you to review the list with everyone in the family, not so much to identify OCD correctly as to bring everyone along in doing the program in a supportive and mutually pleasing way. Remember, a central brainpower tool is to remind yourself that there's almost nothing more important than recovering from the illness we call OCD. Be serious and make getting rid of OCD a value for the entire family.

How a therapist can help: When children have a hard time articulating their triggers, obsessions, compulsions, and fear temperatures, and if you are having difficulty changing your view of OCD, a therapist can be a big help in mapping OCD. Some OCD symptoms that involve aggressive urges (such as stabbing a family member with a knife), sexual issues (such as incest or homosexuality), or morality (such as cheating at school) are tough for some people to talk about. Therapists are specifically trained in interview methods that will avoid blaming or embarrassing children or parents, and they can help everyone compile accurate information efficiently.

Also, OCD is sometimes extremely complex, meaning that you end up needing a map of contamination fears, religious worries, and "just so" rituals, in addition to a bunch of things that your child can't even mention. Or in some cases a child just won't budge from "It's all zeroes—no problem" or "It's all 10s—too hard." Kids almost always take this stance because they're afraid that they'll have to do an EX/RP task that is really too hard, but sometimes just pointing this out isn't enough to make acceptance of and relaxing about OCD possible. If these descriptions seem to apply to your child and making a map begins to seem like an endless task, or if you have a nagging suspicion that the map isn't complete but can't be sure what's missing, talk to a trained therapist. This map really is critical to the success of the rest of the program.

Reward Your Child for Progress Made

If you're finding it really difficult not to take charge of the program, here's a great place for you to channel your efforts. It's certainly important for your child to learn how to reinforce his own self-worth by internalizing self-recognition for victories against OCD. But your new role as coach and cheerleader gives you a natural opportunity to support this effort externally.

You can do this, first, by modeling. If you say "Way to go!" often enough and with enough sincere and close attention to true wins against OCD (rather than indiscriminate, insincere flattery), your child will begin to understand on a deeper level how much you really value her accomplishments and will begin to congratulate herself.

As for recording wins against OCD, pull out all the creative stops. Get some new markers and bright poster board. If it works for you, look for stickers that will appeal to your child's particular interests, from dinosaurs to sports to fashion, and use them for a star chart. Make the chart with your child, turning it into a memorably fun and positive project of its own.

As to setting up a reward system, just keep an open mind. Try not to look at these rewards as bribery. You're not trying to cajole your child to resist OCD but simply rewarding the child for the very hard work that resistance requires. After all, he's got even more homework and chores than before. Be sure to come up with rewards that fit into your family culture. You may not believe in giving food as rewards, but little treats can be a quick and simple type of reward for a young child, whether it's a lollipop or a snack-size bag of crackers or cookies.

Obviously, you'll have to be involved in devising the reward system, especially for the youngest children. Sit down with your child and figure out what is important to the child: Choosing the TV program for a half-hour of family viewing time? Getting to set the menu for one dinner a week? An extra bedtime story? Points toward purchase of a new videogame? A little prize or mini-certificate? Whatever serves as a concrete reminder that the child is the author of a new story in which OCD gradually becomes less bossy is appropriate.

When setting up rewards, remember—and remind your child—that the chief reward and motivator is getting rid of OCD. It feels really good to get on top of OCD after so many years on the bottom.

Helping younger kids: Younger kids often need more frequent rewards. Choose some little, tangible prize that you can give out on the spot when the child resists OCD, or give something that can quickly accumulate into something bigger and desirable, such as a full set of inexpensive action figures.

Helping teenagers: The trick here is simply in recognizing that teenagers value different rewards than younger kids or than adults do, with the primary reward (and self-motivator) being getting rid of OCD. Tangible rewards really have to be your teenager's choice, with your job possibly being more to rein in her scope than to pick the category (e.g., a CD for a week's work, not an hour's!).

Taking Stock

Keep an eye on the calendar to help your child stay on track. If 2 weeks have gone by and your child doesn't seem ready for Step 4, you may want to consider talking to a therapist to get you back up to speed.

Step 4: Finishing My Toolkit

WHETHER THE "BATTLE" is a game of tag, a cross-country race, or the drive for good grades, you wouldn't begin without all the proper equipment. In Step 4 of your campaign against OCD, you're going to complete your toolkit so you have everything you need to start conquering the illness. You've got your brainpower tools from Step 3 and a map that shows where, when, and how OCD sabotages you. You have a fear thermometer to tell you when to try to resist OCD and when to back off. And you've lined up rewards for all your victories against OCD. Now it's time to add what will become your number-one tool: exposure and response prevention (EX/RP). To put it briefly, here's how it works:

- The *exposure* principle (the EX in EX/RP) says that if you practice hanging in there and staying in contact with a trigger or obsession repeatedly, the obsession and its uncomfortable feelings will go away. For example, if you were afraid of heights, you would go one step up a 10-step ladder 10 times, get comfortable with that, then take two steps up 10 times and get comfortable with that, and then keep on going to the top of the ladder.
- The *response prevention* principle (the RP in EX/RP) says that exposure will get rid of an obsession and the discomfort it causes you only if you don't do any rituals that OCD usually makes you do. If you bail out mid-task (come down the ladder before getting used to the height) or do your rituals (the equivalent of coming down the ladder), exposure won't work. In fact, it is worse than that: Bailing out (giving in to OCD) once you've committed to an EX/RP task strongly reinforces the brain's tendency to hiccup.

So how do we make sure you go into EX/RP with your eyes open and come out successful? By giving you a toolkit that puts you in charge of selecting tasks from the work zone, where you already know you can win against OCD. Armed with the EX/RP tool to target symptoms in the work zone, you'll be ready in this step for a trial run against OCD before beginning the full-scale effort to eliminate OCD from your life. From here on the real fight against OCD begins, in the form of CBT work that we will call simply "tasks" from now on.

At this stage, if you're like most kids and parents, you hope EX/RP will work, but down deep inside you don't really believe it will. After all, you've had OCD for a long time. After Step 4, however, you will be a believer. And though it will not always be easy, 3 months from now, if you work hard, there's a really good chance that you can be well again.

The Game Plan for Step 4

Once you've done the reading and other preparation listed under "Get Ready," follow the instructions for Step 4. Plan to spend about 3 to 4 days on this trial run in resisting OCD and then take stock of how you're doing. At this point a little more than a week should have passed since you started the program. *If the trial tasks in this step don't leave you feeling confident and eager to keep forging ahead, take another few days and choose another trial task with a lower fear temperature to practice. If you're not feeling like you're on track toward having the upper hand against OCD, you may need help from a therapist.* Post the "Getting Stronger Every Day" chart where you'll see it easily, and on it check off the completion of each day's work.

Get Ready

Last week you did a lot of detailed detective work. Let's take a look at what you turned up: When you tried talking back to OCD, what happened? In which situations did it get easier to boss OCD around over the week, and in which did it stay the same or get even harder? When you told yourself that maybe you could handle this much discomfort this one time when you were feeling that you had to do a ritual, in what cases did the fear thermometer go up? Where did it go down? Which brainpower techniques helped you most? Did refusing to buy into OCD's threats help you avoid any rituals? How often were you able to let OCD float by without focusing your attention on it? In what situations were you able to do this? How well did relaxing and quietly letting OCD float by without resistance work, as compared with powerfully telling OCD to buzz off? In what order did you find yourself using these tools most successfully?

Talk over these questions with your parents to see if they have any ideas. Jot down a new script or list of reminders on your brainpower card if you found yourself using only certain of the tools or using them in a different order from the one you originally wrote. This will be your brainpower routine for the future, or at least for the time being.

Now take a look at the notes you jotted about the triggers, obsessions, and compulsions in your chart. If you haven't used them to change the fear temperature as needed in your chart, do it now, so that you'll be able to accurately identify OCD symptoms that fall into the work zone.

Post the summary of Step 4 from the back of this book where you'll see it often, to remind you of what you're going to do the rest of this week. Also keep your OCD symptom chart (map) handy. It doesn't have to be pasted up on your wall where everyone can see it if you don't want to do that, but it should be easy to see and reach, with a pencil nearby for jotting notes or making any changes you want to make this week.

Reread Chapter 4 if you need to review how EX/RP works in more detail or if you need a refresher course on the types of tasks that it involves. Or ask your parents to review this for you.

Get Going

Fill In the Work Zone

You've probably heard the advice "pick your battles" before—maybe when your mother was encouraging you not to argue about every single chore you're assigned or when you were complaining about a million things that your little sister does to bug you. This wise advice is based on a couple of well-known facts:

1. Attacking an enemy everywhere at once is likely to stretch your forces too thin and increase the chances that you'll lose all the battles (and thus the whole war).
2. The surest way to get beaten up is to pick fights that you're bound to lose.

The *work zone* is the battleground on which you have a really good chance of being 100% successful in beating OCD. It's the place where winning over OCD will give you confidence that you can get rid of OCD in a big way. The work zone is where you're going to start trying homework assignments for directly resisting OCD, so you need to figure out exactly which of the OCD symptoms that you listed in your chart fall into this zone. Why is this important? Because it is much easier to convert partial success (tasks from the work zone) to 100% success than it is to convert zero success (tasks above the work zone) to 100% success, and it is 100% success that is our goal. Less than that just serves to reinforce OCD. To make your brain stop hiccupping, you need to win each and every time. Here's what belongs in your work zone:

- *Symptoms (hiccups) with fear temperatures of 2-3.* In Step 2 you learned that the symptoms with a fear temperature of 2-3 are the ones where you could beat OCD more than half of the time. Any symptoms in your chart that have a fear temperature of 2-3 definitely belong in your work zone. But they may not be the only actions or situations that belong there.
- *Symptoms (hiccups) with fear temperatures of 4-5 for which you resisted some part of the ritual some of the time.* Think about the successes you had in talking back to OCD over the past week. Where did you successfully resist OCD at least some of the time? Some of these belong in your work zone, too, even if their fear temperature is a 4 or, very rarely, a 5. Pull out your symptom chart and look at the group of hiccups that fall together between fear temperatures 2 and 3, maybe 4. If you have more than one "flavor" of OCD, you may have work zones in each of those groups of hiccups on your chart. How did you do in these situations last week? Were you able to resist performing the ritual at least half of the time for these? If so, they all belong in your work zone.
- *Symptoms (hiccups) with a higher fear temperature that you can break down so that they have a lower fear temperature.* Now look closely at the other symptoms. Can you break them down into parts so that there is a work zone within each? Let's say OCD makes you wash your hands five times, starting with your right thumb and moving to the pinkie on the right hand, then doing the left, after you touch the sink in your bathroom. Maybe you've assigned touching a sink without performing this ritual a temperature of 6. This temperature keeps the action of touching the sink out of the work zone—unless you can, for example, wash your hands without doing each finger in order sometimes. Maybe just violating the one rule that OCD sets is a 3 on the temperature chart. If you can do that, then maybe the task that falls into the work zone is washing your hands the same number of times but in any order after touching the sink.

Now do the same exercise for all your OCD symptoms above the work zone. What you want to do is get a sense of where you already can break the rules that OCD sets. This means not just guessing but figuring out what you've actually been able to do in the last couple of days. Look back at the notes you've been taking if that helps.

For example, don't just guess whether you could touch the sink and wash less. Ask yourself, "During the past week, what is the shortest time that OCD got me washing? Was there a time that I broke the rule about which fingers to wash in a row?" "How about the time I went to school when I wasn't sure about my right sock? I bet I can leave one sock a little off this week." "Was there a time that I didn't check the locks, the oven, the toaster plug, my dad to be sure he was OK?" "How about skipping counting, or not going back if I get out of order?"

Maybe you noticed that in some situations—perhaps when you were caught up with something else—you resisted performing a ritual without ever thinking about it. Maybe you didn't have to wash your hands after touching the water fountain when you were rushing to get to class on time before an important test. Or maybe just letting OCD float by when it told you that your mother was going to get sick if you brought germs into the house after soccer practice made it possible for you to open the door with your bare hand rather than using your jacket sleeve to grasp the doorknob. Believe it—you are already winning over OCD a lot of the time. You just need to recognize it and to convert this to 100% of the time. Use your life experiences to identify work zone tasks, and you're well on the way to defying OCD.

Here's an example:

Action/situation/trigger (if any)	Obsession	Compulsion	Temp. (1–10)
Touch toilet and then eat lunch.	I'll get sick from eating germy food.	Wash hands for 5 minutes.	10
Touch sink and then eat lunch.	Same	Same	6
Touch door to bathroom with hand rather than shirt and then eat lunch.	Same	Same	4
Touch door to bathroom with hand rather than shirt and then eat lunch.	Same	Wash hands for as long as needed, but skip little finger of left hand.	3

Owen's fear thermometer will go up to 6 if he touches the sink without washing his hands for 5 minutes before lunch. But because of the times he remembered he was able to talk back to OCD or let it float by last week, he figured he could lower the fear temperature to 5 if he washed all but his pinkie for 1 minute, to 4 if he washed his whole hands for 1 minute, to 3 if he washed for 2 minutes, and to 2 if he washed for 3 minutes. He could make it more manageable if he just went into the bathroom without using his shirt to touch the door, and even more manageable by washing for as long as necessary but skipping one finger. All of the tasks with fear temperatures of 2–4, and possibly even the one he assigned a 5, belong in his work zone.

Another example:

Action/situation/trigger (if any)	Obsession	Compulsion	Temp. (1–10)
Put on socks in the morning without making sure they're balanced.	I'll feel nervous and upset that something is wrong all day.	Spend 20 minutes balancing socks and asking Mom if they look even.	9

Sally said she couldn't spend her usual 20 minutes balancing her socks on a couple of mornings during the past week, and judging by her experience when that happened, she would rate balancing her socks for only 2 minutes a 6, for 6 minutes a 5, for 8 minutes a 4, for 10 minutes a 3, and spending the full 20 minutes but without asking Mom to assure her that they were even a 2.

Most kids can actually divide up each basic symptom on their chart to make a list of EX/RP tasks for that symptom that have fear temperatures ranging from 1 to 10. See if this works for you. You pick one symptom from your hiccup chart and arrange specific tasks to tackle like a ladder, then pick items 1–4 to work on at any given time. You can keep revising your task lists as you work your way through the steps of the program.

Because some hiccups are triggered by something that goes on around you or that you run into and some just pop up on their own, there are two different ways to do EX/RP. You can tackle a task when a hiccup is triggered, or you can purposely put yourself in the position of having a hiccup so that you can practice dealing with it without doing a ritual. Some of each of these two types of tasks appear in the following lists. We'll get into this difference more in Step 5.

Example of EX/RP Task List for HIV Contamination

10. Shake hands with person with AIDS.
9. Talk to person with AIDS.
8. Go to hospice where persons with HIV die and touch door, sit in furniture.
7. Go to place where a person with HIV might hang out.
6. Talk to and touch someone who works with patients with HIV.
5. Eat in a public place and use a restroom without washing.
4. Watch a DVD about AIDS.
3. Google on HIV/AIDS.
2. Read an article about HIV or AIDS in *Newsweek*.
1. Talk about fear of HIV with a friend or family member.

Example of EX/RP Task List for One Dirty Object with Harm to Self

10. Wear dirty shirt; don't wash.
9. Wear shirt next to dirty shirt; don't wash.
8. Wear shirt two shirts away from dirty shirt; don't wash.
7. Touch dirty shirt; don't wash.
6. Touch shirt next to dirty shirt; don't wash.
5. Touch shirt two shirts away from dirty shirt; don't wash.
4. Wear clean shirt in same closet as dirty shirt; don't wash.
3. Put dirty shirt in closet; don't wash.
2. Put dirty shirt near but not in closet; don't wash.
1. Wash dirty shirt, but don't wash hands after.

Example of EX/RP Task List for Checking

10. Leave oven on and leave house for 1 hour.
9. Leave toaster plugged in and leave house.
8. Don't check door locks at night.
7. Don't check window locks at night.
6. Check that toaster plug is out once only.
5. Check front door lock once only.
4. Check that oven isn't on once only.
3. Don't call Dad at work to ask if he locked car.
2. Don't check bike lock during recess.
1. Don't try to remember and rehash locking bike lock.

Example of EX/RP Task List for "Just So" Arranging

10. Wear mismatched clothes that are all rumpled up.
 9. Leave shirttail hanging out.
 8. Let pencil on left side of desk sit sideways.
 7. Don't even up socks when getting dressed.
 6. Let socks get uneven during day without making them even.
 5. Walk through doors at school off center.
 4. Walk through doors at home off center.
 3. Don't straighten silverware before eating.
 2. Don't touch left and then right side of plate before eating.
 1. Sit crooked on couch.

Example of EX/RP Task List for Moral Scrupulosity (Cheating)

10. Look at another student's paper during a test.
 9. Don't ask teacher if somehow I might have cheated.
 8. Look around class and watch other students taking tests.
 7. Don't make intentional mistake to prove I didn't cheat.
 6. Don't inspect test answers to see if somehow I might have cheated.
 5. Imagine cheating on a test.
 4. Talk to other students about cheating.
 3. Make list of 10 reasons cheating is a good idea.
 2. Label worry about cheating as OCD.
 1. Do math homework problems without checking answers.

Example of EX/RP Task List for Religious Scrupulosity (Praying in Response to Sexual Thought)

10. Look at porn site on Internet without praying.
 9. Look at *Playboy* without praying.
 8. Have sexual thoughts without praying.
 7. Write down sex words without praying.
 6. Write down sex words, but violate praying rules (hard).
 5. Write down sex words, but violate praying rules (moderately hard).
 4. Write down sex words, but violate praying rules (easy).
 3. Talk to minister about praying and OCD.
 2. Cut down praying repetitions (hard).
 1. Cut down praying repetitions (easy).

Example of EX/RP Task List for Counting (4 is good, 7 is bad number)

10. No counting all day.
9. Count to 7 for 1 minute each hour.
8. Do 100 math problems, each of which has a lot of 7s in it.
7. Do 100 math problems with one 7 in each.
6. Wash three, not four, times.
5. Brush hair seven, not four, times.
4. Use number 7 in conversation.
3. Write the number 7 one hundred times.
2. Read a math book and underline the number 7 7 x 7 times.
1. Say "seven" to yourself 100 times.

Example of EX/RP Task List for Hoarding

10. Throw away old notebooks.
9. Don't check to see if I still have old notebooks.
8. Throw away boxes for action figures.
7. Don't inventory action figures.
6. Don't check trash can outside for "lost" objects.
5. Throw out old papers in closet.
4. Empty trash can in bedroom without checking.
3. Throw out scrap paper from today.
2. Make a list of all the bad things hoarding does to you and throw it away.
1. Make a list of hoarded objects and throw it away.

Did you beat OCD on any triggers that you ranked near 8–10 on the fear thermometer last week? If so, you've probably assigned these a temperature that's too high. Try lowering the number to see whether any way you modify a ritual puts the symptom in the work zone. But don't go too far. If you were able to resist something you had assigned an 8 once last week, you might give it a 6 or 7 now; don't give it a 4 or 5. The last thing you want is to be overconfident and as a result set yourself up. You should know, however, that this is exactly what will happen later in the program. When you knock off what's in the work zone, the tasks above it will migrate downward into the work zone, meaning that they will become easier without your having to do anything to make it so.

Remember, we call this a *work zone* because its territory isn't controlled by either you or OCD; you win there sometimes, and OCD wins there sometimes. The object is for you to start to win there all the time, and that's also why we call this the work zone. It's from this list of triggers that you will be choosing symptoms to work on, to get them across that border and into your territory.

As we said before, what's in the work zone will shift as you work through this program. This fact has two important implications. First, things that are above the work zone will come down to an easier temperature automatically as you get better at beating OCD. What is now an 8 will be a 4 or 5 in a few weeks without your having to do anything at all. Second, it is critical that you and your parents not try to tackle things that are too hard. You've had OCD for a while now, and it will profit you to be patient and kind with yourselves and each other for OCD symptoms that are too high on the OCD symptom chart to tackle yet.

So now that you've reviewed all the ways you can add to your work zone, make a new chart, again in temperature order. Make a few copies (photocopies are great) of this chart. On one of them, circle your work zone in a bright highlighter. This way you'll be able to focus on what your targets are for the coming week. As each week of the program ends, you can pull out a new photocopy of your chart, change the fear thermometer ratings to reflect your victories, and circle a new group of triggers to highlight your new work zone.

The symptom (hiccup) chart with the work zones circled for the sample map we've been using so far is shown on the next page.

There are other tasks this boy could list in his work zone, too. Because getting the curtains closed evenly was right on the border of the work zone, he decided to break it down into two different tasks. One was just closing the curtains once and then leaving them that way. That task still had a fear temperature of 4, sometimes even 5. But another task could be limiting the number of times he adjusted the curtains to three times. After that, he'd just go to bed and start reading his book. He gave this task a 2 and put it in the work zone.

This boy also had two hiccups in his chart that had temperatures of 6. He really didn't like covering doorknobs with his sleeve or a tissue, because he thought other kids and his family noticed him doing it, and he really wanted to be rid of OCD here. So he decided to break down that symptom into a separate mini-task list so he could start working on it right away. Here's what it looked like:

EX/RP Task List for Touching Doorknobs

10. Use bare hands to open doors.
 9. Touch other doorknobs with only one or two fingers.
 8. Open door of family car with bare hands.
 7. Open other doors at home with bare hands.
 6. Open my own bedroom door with bare hands.
 5. Have Mom grasp doorknob with my hand over hers while she opens the door.
 4. Let someone else open doors, but then brush my bare arm against doorknob.

Action/situation/trigger (if any)	Obsession	Compulsion	Temp. (1–10)
WASHING			
Touching toilet	"I'll get germy and make Mom sick."	Avoid touching toilet or wash hands 5 times.	10
Using friend's bathroom	"I'll get their family's germs and make my family sick."	Avoid visiting for long enough to need the bathroom.	8
Touching my mouth with my fingers	"I'll get sick and die from germs on my hands."	Wash hands every time my fingers touch my mouth.	6
Touching doorknobs	"I'll get people's germs and get sick."	Use shirt, tissue, or coat to hold doorknobs.	6
Petting the dog	"The dog's germs will spread and make everyone sick."	Pet dog with gloves on or wash hands 5 times.	3
Walking by dog after shower	Ditto	Don't walk within 6 feet of the dog.	1–2
ORDERING OR ARRANGING			
Getting dressed for school	"I have to make sure my socks are evened up."	Even up socks over and over until they feel right. Ask Mom whether they look straight.	5
Ditto	"I have to make sure my hair is combed evenly."	Comb hair over and over until it looks right in the mirror.	5
Going to bed	"The curtains need to be closed evenly so they meet right in the center of the window."	Pull curtains closed, step back to check them, then adjust them over and over.	3–4
Ditto	"My covers have to be folded over evenly when Mom tucks me in."	Mom has to keep tucking them in until they feel right to me.	3
Getting dressed for school	"My watch has to be right in the middle of my wrist."	Don't wear watch or adjust it on my wrist till it looks right.	1–2

3. Let someone else open doors, but then touch the person's hand briefly.
2. Cover doorknobs with sleeve, but then touch door near doorknob with bare hand.
1. Cover doorknobs with sleeve, but hold on to doorknob for 5 seconds.

At this point you might have work zone tasks from three different sources, just like this boy: some symptoms circled on your symptom chart; a symptom rated 4 that you've broken down so that part of it comes into the work zone, because you can beat OCD sometimes that way; and some tasks in the work zone from a task list you've made up for one symptom that you want to be sure to get rid of eventually. If it's easier for you to see these all together, you can put them on another blank copy of your symptom chart, like the one shown on page 170.

Especially when they've written up separate EX/RP lists for specific symptoms, however, many kids like to keep those separate and just think of them as "hiccup ladders" that they start to work their way up over the next several weeks.

Complete the Toolkit

The goal here is simply to pack up your gear, making sure you have everything and that it's all in working order and that you know how to use it before you set out for your trial battle. You now have several tools for combating OCD:

- Your brainpower strategies for talking back to OCD (Chapters 5, 6, and 7).
- Your fear thermometer for gauging when you're making progress or about to head into trouble (Chapter 6).
- Your updated OCD symptom chart (map; this chapter).
- Your transition or work zone map (part of your symptom chart or some separate EX/RP task lists; this chapter).
- Your reward system for efforts you make to boss OCD back (Chapter 7).

You can think of all of these as your weapons or your tools. Some kids think of these skillful coping strategies as military weapons in the war against OCD or as the instruments in a doctor's bag or as the tools on a carpenter's belt. However you view them, they're what you need to get the job done, and now is the time to make sure that they work and that you know how to use them.

- Do you feel pretty comfortable talking back to OCD at this point? You can practice this at any time but will definitely need to use it during your trial task and all the tasks to come. It's easy to talk calmly about OCD when you're not in the middle of an attack. For this reason, you need to practice talking back to OCD

Your Work Zone

Action/situation/trigger (if any)	Obsession	Compulsion	Temp. (1–10)
WASHING			
Petting the dog	"The dog's germs will spread and make everyone sick."	Pet dog with gloves on or wash hands 5 times.	3
Walking by dog after shower	Ditto	Don't walk within 6 feet of the dog.	1–2
ORDERING OR ARRANGING			
Going to bed	"My covers have to be folded over evenly when Mom tucks me in."	Mom has to keep tucking them in until they feel right to me.	3
Ditto	"The curtains need to be closed evenly so they meet right in the center of the window."	Adjust curtains no more than three times before getting into bed.	2
Getting dressed for school	"My watch has to be right in the middle of my wrist."	Don't wear watch or adjust it on my wrist till it looks right.	1–2
Touching doorknobs			
		Let someone else open doors, but then touch the person's hand briefly.	3
		Cover doorknobs with sleeve, but then touch door near doorknob with bare hand.	2
		Cover doorknob with sleeve, but hold on to doorknob for 5 seconds.	1

when it is yelling obsessions at you, which it most definitely will do when you start resisting in the next steps. Talking back under OCD's pressure will help you lower the fear thermometer, which will always be your goal.

• How accurate is your fear thermometer? All the review of the Step 3 work that you just completed should give you a pretty good idea of whether you're using the fear thermometer appropriately.

• Have you gotten in the habit of giving yourself rewards (or getting them from your parents) after each time you try to boss back OCD? If not, spend another day or two on this until it becomes the automatic wrap-up following each effort you make.

• Is your brainpower routine from Step 3 in good order? Have you tinkered with it so that it works best for you?

Before you move on to the next goal for this step, rehearse your brainpower routine, either alone or with a parent or therapist, until you can call it into play on command, as quickly and smoothly as you'd come up with answers to why you haven't done your chores or what happened to the paper that was supposed to be on your teacher's desk this morning. Make sure that your brainpower reminder card is filled out and ready to use when you start your EX/RP task.

Practice a Trial EX/RP Task

Give yourself a pat on the back: You've completed your basic preparation and you're now armed and ready to try your first on-purpose foray into territory occupied by OCD. Look back and think about how much has changed in just a few days— you now know what OCD is; you can talk to yourself about OCD in a way that makes you feel better, not worse; you have a good road map of what to do; and your family is on your side. Now you are ready to boss back OCD in one small part of the work zone. The goal here is not to hammer one OCD symptom into the ground, though that will happen, but to practice everything you've learned so far together, so that next week you can start moving up your list of OCD symptoms, nailing OCD one or two at a time.

The next few days are just a trial run to make sure that you have it all ready to go. OK, here we go.

First, you need to choose a symptom from your chart. A broad range of temperatures are represented on your symptom chart, but you need to pick a symptom from the work zone—a 2, or, at highest, a 3. Look at your 2s and 3s and pick one that you're sure you can tackle with relative ease. This should be one that you were able to resist without much difficulty more than half the time last week when it came up. Up to now you weren't really doing an EX/RP task on purpose, so if you can resist half the time, you should easily be able to convert a 2 to a 0 now that you have a completed toolkit. The point here is simply to practice using your toolkit, so which symptom you pick doesn't really matter. It just has to be really easy. Once you've chosen a symptom, find a quiet time and place to see how it all works and give it a go.

Try it first in imagination. Let's say you've chosen going into the house via the back door without using your sleeve to turn the doorknob. Usually you would use your sleeve to avoid bringing the outdoor "germs" into the house with you and making your family sick, and you've noticed that over the past week you beat OCD about 9 out of 10 times, either because you're in a big hurry to get in and don't think about what OCD might say or because you talk back to OCD and say something like "Not this time, OCD." Or maybe you just say "Oh, there's old Stupid again" when OCD tells you to watch out for germs on the doorknob, and you let OCD float by, left outside while you go in. So you've assigned this trigger a 2, and it's in the work zone, right on the border of territory you already control.

Picture yourself going into the house. As you see yourself approaching the door, ready to go in, ask yourself how high your fear thermometer has gone up. It may go up to a 2 right away, or maybe, because you're just imagining the trigger, you can keep it at a 1. Now picture yourself grasping the doorknob with your bare hand. Using everything you have in your toolkit, talk back to OCD, but keep on holding on to that doorknob. Don't let go and don't give in to the urge to grab your sleeve to use it to turn the knob. Imagine staying right there until your fear comes down, to a 1 if it started at 2, to 0 if it started at 1. In your mind, don't use your sleeve or let go of the doorknob until your fear has gone down to that level. And, of course, don't wash once you're inside the house.

OK, now that you've practiced it in imagination, do it for real. Go find the doorknob (or whatever your task is), and don't let OCD get the better of you. Touch the doorknob repeatedly with your bare hand until it gets boring, go inside, and don't wash. Use all the tools in your toolkit as you need to, until your fear thermometer goes down from 2 to 1 or from 1 to 0.

Hey! You did it. You've beaten OCD, and you should give yourself a big hug. But before you do, just remember for a moment how many months or years OCD has been around, and be proud of how far you've come in just a few days. You've got plenty of hard work ahead, surely, but even so the edge is now yours. Congratulations!

Now, for the next week, whether you use this symptom or choose another one that's a 2 or 3 within your work zone, practice exposing yourself to this trigger once every day. Twice is even better. Do it for real. If it's a trigger that you can, and often do, avoid, then practice by choosing to face that trigger. Do it at a set time each day. If it's something you can't avoid, pick a window of time during which you'll try to resist it once, or, if it seems possible, try to resist every time you're exposed to it. *But be aware of your fear temperature at all times. If trying to resist more than once sends your fear temperature soaring, back off and stick to once a day for the week.*

While you're doing the trial task, rate your anxiety using the fear thermometer every few minutes throughout the task. If you think it will help you keep track, you can record your fear temperature on the form on the following page. Right before you start the task, you're likely to feel some anxiety or discomfort in anticipation. Immediately use your brainpower tools, the ones you wrote on your 3 × 5 card. Talk back to OCD as soon as you feel the urge to perform your usual ritual, and resist performing the ritual until your fear temperature comes down to 0. Don't quit until you get down to a 0 or you'll let OCD win at the last minute. After you finish the task, write down which brainpower tools you used if you're using the Task Record forms.

Keep your Task Record forms in a folder or a drawer until the end of the step. If you think it will be helpful to you, use them to see how you did.

Amy, age 8, chose to target a really simple task from her work zone because she was afraid that she'd blow it. With her mom holding the door open, she walked one foot into the bathroom at McDonald's and walked right out again. This was a big deal as for years she'd been unable to use the bathroom at restaurants. Guess what? "It was easy," Amy said.

Pedro, 15, had tapping and touching rituals for getting in and out of chairs and going through doors. He picked a task that involved going through a door at home and touching just one side, not both. This was an easy task as mostly he skipped this door anyway. At first, he was mad about doing the extra homework, but it was so much fun that he did it laughing for 30 minutes and then, just for the heck of it, did another 30 minutes with several doors, not touching or tapping at all. His comment: "I am the greatest." Mom hadn't seen him that happy in a long time.

Doug, a 9-year-old boy with ADHD and OCD, just couldn't stick out the EX/RP task—not because he didn't want to but because ADHD got in the way. His mom took him to his pediatrician, and they adjusted his medication. After this, Doug had no trouble throwing out scraps of paper and not picking them back out of the trash.

TASKS

_____

_____

_____

_____

BRAINPOWER TOOLS

_____

_____

_____

_____

Target/ date/ time	Start temp.	1 min.	2 min.	5 min.	10 min.	15 min.	20 min.	25 min.	30 min.

Five-year-old Allen had repeating rituals involving numbers. He chose to put his socks on four times on the left and five times on the right instead of five times on both sides. His mom sat there with him checking off the number of repeats on a piece of paper and listening to Allen telling stories and jokes. The next day it was four and four, then three and three, then two and two, and then that one was gone. "Amazingly easy," said Mom. Allen wanted a hamburger.

Twelve-year-old Danielle had very complex and time-consuming washing and grooming rituals that came from OCD telling her that she had to have her hair and makeup "just so" or she'd have a "bad day." Danielle chose to use a different kind of lipstick than OCD usually wanted. The first time OCD got nasty, and she gave in and put the regular lipstick on so she wouldn't have to start the whole sequence again and be late for school. Although her mom wanted her to try something easier, the next day she vowed not to give in to OCD, and she didn't. She had a really good day, too! Even more amazing, Danielle went from 3 to 4 hours in the bathroom every day to less than 30 minutes within a month. "That's less than my prissy friends," she said with a laugh.

Taking Stock

About 2 weeks—and no more than 3—should have passed since you started the program, and you've reached an important milestone once you've completed Step 4. Use the OCD scale and graph one more time and take a look at the difference between your ratings now and when you started out. The change might not be huge yet, but it sure will be noticeable. It's only going to get better in the next several weeks, so let's keep going.

Step 4: Instructions for Parents

THIS STEP MARKS an important turning point in the program. Step 4 is the last preliminary, preparatory step. During the next few days your child will be adding to his kit the last of the fundamental tools to be used throughout the subsequent steps. He will figure out where OCD has a hold of him much but not all of the time and will use this knowledge to begin to resist OCD skillfully. When he sees that he really can beat OCD at its own game, you'll find that he'll be very motivated to continue chipping away at OCD over the coming weeks.

The Game Plan for Step 4

This is an important turning point for you, too. So far your main goal has been to shift your attitude toward OCD in the same way that your child has and to interact differently with your child about OCD. We've cautioned you not to be worried about resisting OCD in the first few steps, because this program will work best if your child is empowered to take charge. If your child has completed Steps 1–3 successfully, you've obviously been a terrific coach and cheerleader. You should plan on continuing in that role for the rest of the program. Here, though, you may need to exercise a little more supervision or direct involvement, especially with preadolescents. All the tools need to be in place and in good working order if your child is to succeed in eliminating OCD in the following steps. She needs to have an accurate "map" of her OCD symptoms so she can choose to work on the symptoms that will allow her to make headway and motivate her to continue. If she stalls by focusing on tasks that are too easy, she'll lose that motivation. Failure due to targeting tasks that are too hard too soon will play right into OCD's hands and decrease motivation to stay with the program. So, although we still ask you to remember that your child is ultimately the only one who can resist OCD, during this step you need to be especially vigilant as to whether your child has in fact achieved what the program requires before moving on. And don't forget, if your child really hasn't made any inroads at all into OCD, and she's been working at the program for 3 weeks, it is definitely time to call in a therapist.

There's probably nothing more important to your child's success with EX/RP tasks than *not* bailing out. That's why it's essential for him to pick tasks that are really in the work zone. Bailing out on tasks only reinforces OCD. So be prepared to review your child's chosen tasks carefully and then also to coach your child to use all the brainpower techniques at his disposal to tolerate the anxiety of the exposure. I know I'm asking you to tread a fine line. You can't take over the program, or the habituation that is supposed to occur from doing the tasks successfully won't have a chance to happen. But if you stay out of it entirely, your child may not get needed support to hang in there. So be gentle, feel your way, and watch your child's reaction. Is your coaching helping him let OCD float by, or is it making him shift his focus from the task at hand to his competence at it? If it's the latter, you'll probably sense it in his emotional reaction. Starting to worry about whether they're "failing" almost always makes kids more anxious, and you want to see the fear temperature going down—not through the child's avoidance of the "hiccup" but by his sticking out the exposure for long enough to make the temperature drop.

Get Ready

Before going on, review Chapter 4, as well as the preceding kids' section of this chapter, so that you are clear about what's required: defining the work zone, picking a trial EX/RP task from the work zone, and seeing that task through to a successful completion using the brainpower tools that you and your child have learned so far.

No shortcuts in this step. Be sure to ask if your child needs any help gathering the charts and forms required to follow the instructions. Make a habit of asking at the end of each day whether she has checked off her completed assignments on the "Getting Stronger Every Day" form. Offer congratulations and rewards when you notice any successes and ask your child if you're catching them all.

Be sure to have the review discussion described in the kids' section and listen carefully to what your child has to say about his experience during Step 3. What went well? What didn't go well and needs further attention? You may want to remind him that successful people spend much more time working on what doesn't go well than on what comes easily and that when he gets it right it will feel really good. Have the symptom chart handy during this discussion to make sure that any necessary additions or revisions are made, either by your child or with your help. It's much easier to keep updating this chart frequently than to have to retrace your steps and try to figure out days after the fact what and where things have changed.

Get Going

Fill In the Work Zone

Even if your son or daughter is old enough to work out the work zone alone, you should review what he or she has come up with to make sure it doesn't contradict your observations. Some children get overconfident and tend to rank symptoms too low or too high on the fear thermometer. We call too low "faking good," which is another way of saying "It's so easy, I don't have to do it." Too high is "faking hard," which is another way of saying "It's too hard for me to do it." If you get all 1s or all 10s, you've got this problem, which basically reflects avoidance of the program out of fear that the person with OCD will have to do impossible exposure and response prevention tasks. If you notice this tendency in your child's chart, gently ask your child how often he or she beat OCD in those areas last week. Remind your child that only those triggers that the child beat more than half of the time should get a 2 or 3. Be sure that he and you understand that the only targets for EX/RP that are OK to tackle on purpose reside in the work zone. Though harder tasks may show up in the work zone as the week goes by, there's no pressure to go higher.

Whether or not you see any signs that your child is trying to do too much too fast, encourage your child to be patient. Remind the child that this is a learning process. Just as he didn't become a piano virtuoso after three lessons or she didn't make the varsity swim team at age 10, your child won't beat OCD all at once.

Do the same for yourself. Always remember that your role is to serve as coach and cheerleader, not to scold or be the chief operating officer. Actually, the program is the coach, and you're the assistant coach. Follow the program and you'll be all right. When your child talks about having resisted OCD, be sure to offer compliments. It's often better, however, to reinforce the child's feelings than to reinforce the performance. Say "That must have made you feel really good" or "It must have felt great to realize that you could beat OCD more than you thought" instead of "Good job!" Children who tend to be self-critical, which includes many kids with OCD, need to be reminded that it's not achievement per se that they're after but the confidence and serenity that come from knowing they have power over OCD. It's that confidence that will keep them going toward the next step. You want them to focus on that, not the "score" for the week.

Helping younger kids: Younger kids will need parental help in filling in the work zone. You'll have to start a dialogue to review last week's work and see which symptoms really fall into the fear temperature range of 2–4 or so. Your child also may be one of the few who just doesn't get the idea of a work zone. If those terms only confuse him, try using a metaphor that embodies the idea captured by the work zone. Maybe your child would like to call it "the soccer field" or the "basketball court" if such terms convey the idea that this is where work is done and battles are won.

Helping teenagers: Be forewarned that many teenagers, even though they hate

OCD and want to get rid of it, don't have much patience with anything that smacks of busy work. They want to get right into the game and forget about all this paperwork. They have enough homework as it is. So you'll have to be particularly careful not to put them on the defensive should you ask about their symptom chart and whether they've defined the work zone. If your teen gets defensive and you suspect she just hasn't done this work, gently remind her that nothing is as important to her as eliminating OCD. Remind her to think about how much better she'll feel and how much more free time she'll have when she doesn't have to deal with OCD anymore. Tell her you understand that this seems like a lot of boring work but that this is important to her as a person and, just as important, to her brain and that therefore she should get on with it.

How a therapist can help: It's important that you agree with your child's assessment of what should be in the work zone. If you don't, but your child (especially a teenager) resists discussing it and revising it with you, you may need to consult a therapist. The trial and all subsequent EX/RP tasks are going to be chosen from this work zone, and it's crucial that they be ones that the child is sure to succeed in. So if you can't seem to get the work zone right, you probably ought to see a therapist to head off the demoralizing possibility of failure on the first trial. It just might be that the child's take on things was right—kids with OCD are, after all, very intelligent—but an uneasy parent will make a poor cheerleader, so it's best to clear up any disagreement before proceeding. Sometimes the child and parents have distinctly different views of how to rank various symptoms. If they can't come to agreement and the disparity seems wide, there might be misunderstanding about how the fear thermometer works. If you and your child disagree widely on the temperature for various symptoms, you may not be there yet and should talk to your therapist or stick with Step 3 for a little longer.

Or there might be such a bad history with OCD or just conflict about house rules that it is impossible to get it together to do the homework required by the program. Where there's little or no giving in to OCD by the family, a teenager who wants to do the program on his own should be allowed to do that. But if the family is tangled up in OCD and you can't all get on the same page, a professional will be necessary.

Complete the Toolkit

Nothing new is necessarily required here. Just ask yourself how confident you are that your child has a good grasp of how to use the tools and skills acquired so far. Running through a rehearsal of the brainpower techniques on your child's card is always a good idea, but don't insist on it if it clearly seems like more work to your child. If possible, turn it into a game. You might say, keeping it light, "Let's see how fast you can name the order you plan use your brainpower techniques." If your child seems to think that would be fun, go for it. If not, just try looking at the card, complimenting her for having it all in order, and then read them out loud, as if for your own benefit.

Practice a Trial EX/RP Task

Depending on what OCD is like and on how well the child has picked up the tools in the toolkit and can use them independently, you may want to help out here either not at all, a little, or a lot. The trick is to figure out which is constructive. First, make sure your child has chosen something that really is a 2 or 3. When kids choose a trigger that actually causes more anxiety than they are admitting, such as a 4 or 5, it may seem manageable when they first imagine exposing themselves to it. But then, when they try it in the real world, their fear can quickly go higher, which very well might make them unable to resist performing the ritual. *It is critical that the task they choose be one that they can succeed at, because failure will make it very hard to persuade the child to go beyond this trial and engage in exposure and response prevention tasks during the rest of the program.* Too easy is much better than too hard! Ask your child if he or she wants you to be around during the daily trials. If so, be sure to praise him for every effort, provide rewards according to the system you've agreed on, and reinforce the child's positive feelings about success.

Use your knowledge of your child, your and your child's preferences, and what you've learned from the program so far to decide on level of involvement. Remember, you can (and should) move more and more into the background as your child internalizes the principles embodied in the toolkit. With middle-school kids, perhaps you'll want to start by being within reach but out of sight, around the corner. Irrespective of the age of your child, encouraging him to keep OCD out in the room as something impersonal and to stay with the program knowing that he's already been successful half the time in this task should help.

The more anxious your child gets, the calmer you should get, so that your child can borrow calmness and confidence from you.

Sometimes it's helpful to find something else to do or just to take fear thermometer readings every few minutes. Watching them go up and then come down can be very interesting.

Thirteen-year-old Gretchen chose to touch her cat and then touch her younger brother. OCD told her that if she did this, he'd get parasites and die. He was pretty sick of being the object of OCD, and Gretchen and her mother had little difficulty in persuading him to take part. Gretchen touched the cat, and she and her brother sat with Mom and watched TV until OCD got bored and left.

Nine-year-old Keisha, whose OCD made her straighten her sheets, pillows, and blanket every night until it felt "just right," chose to straighten everything except her favorite small pink pillow. Her mom, who had to sign off at the end of 30 to 60 minutes of straightening, knew now not to interrupt OCD, as Keisha would have to start over. Keisha asked her to just be there and to read her a story while OCD made its usual fuss and then accepted defeat.

Adam, age 17, had very complex praying and grooming rituals and tics and didn't want anything to do with OCD or with his parents. He preferred videogames, but he also knew that he'd never get to college with OCD in the way. His parents asked him directly what he wanted, and he said that it would help him to know that they trusted him to do the trial EX/RP on his own. He also admitted that it would help him to be held accountable, so he suggested that he simply tell his parents what he was planning and then let them know once each day how it was going. They in turn agreed not to ask, which was a relief to him as he was tired of what he called "prying into my business." The trial task went very well, and they continued with this arrangement for the entire program.

OCD made 12-year-old Jill worry that she might have stabbed her baby sister, Emily, and then made her do a lot of different rituals involving checking and asking her parents and others for reassurance that she hadn't hurt the baby. She had a hard time picking a task. Eventually she decided that she would ask her mother if Emily was OK while her mother held Emily (so she could see) but without her mother answering her. Even though she had rated this a 2–3, it seemed really hard to both her and her mother when they first tried it, and Jill got pretty angry when her mom wouldn't respond. Still, they stuck it out, and it got much easier the second and third time around. This was confidence-inspiring for Jill, who went on with the program more easily afterward.

Hannah, age 7, liked her mom around and found it really helpful if Mom did the EX/RP task first, so she did. Later, they played a game in which Hannah taught Mom to do it, but for the trial EX/RP task, Mom touched the drinking fountain and took a drink, and then Hannah did it.

Helping younger kids: You need to make sure that your child understands and appropriately selects one trial task, and you need to be there to walk your child through it. You can model the task yourself to lead your child through. For example, touch the doorknob and refrain from washing afterward. Then have your child touch the doorknob and refrain from washing. While you're modeling the task, you can even have your child prompt you to hang in there, doing the EX/RP task to completion without bailing, and then do the same for your child. Both of you can use the brainpower tools. Do a little debriefing afterward, talking about what worked well to help your child avoid bailing out and giving the child the opportunity to acknowledge her accomplishment.

Helping teenagers: For high school kids, you might stand by during the trial tasks *if asked*. Unless there's a good reason or your teen wants your help, it shows a lot of confidence in your child to give him the freedom to work through the trial EX/RP task on his own. But participating in debriefing can be useful for kids of any age, just because it helps to solidify which brainpower tools worked and which ones weren't really worth calling into play in this kind of situation.

How a therapist can help: If there is difficulty converging on a trial EX/RP task, especially if you and your child disagree and argue about it, you need the help of a therapist. If trial exposures go nowhere, you've probably not located the work zone properly and will need the help of a therapist to sort out how to break down OCD's requirements for rituals into manageable bits.

Taking Stock

Have a real heart-to-heart talk with your child once she feels like she's finished Step 4. If she's not eager to continue with Step 5, she hasn't truly finished this step, and you need to figure out where things have gone wrong. Don't hesitate to call in a therapist if you're at the end of this step and feel stalled.

Step 5: Beginning to Resist

DAY BY DAY. This is your motto for Step 5. You've completed a trial task, and now you're prepared to take on OCD in the work zone a little at a time.

Kids who do trial tasks as you just did report a wide variety of experiences. Were your efforts to defeat OCD a resounding success? A disappointing setback? Something in between? The important thing to take from your experiences during Step 4 is that none should be considered failures in any way. At the very least, your trial task should have left you with information you can use to make more inroads into the work zone than you were able to manage last week—sort of like a scouting mission. But don't be surprised if it turns out that you did a lot better than you think you did. Read on to find out how this might or might not be true for you.

The Game Plan for Step 5

Once you've done the preparation listed under "Get Ready," follow the instructions for Step 5, planning to spend about 3 to 4 weeks on this step. This period will be your first real effort to bring to bear what you've learned in your battle with OCD. Post your "Getting Stronger Every Day" form somewhere visible to you and check off the work you've done each day. After 2 weeks, take stock. If all went well, you'll start working on other symptoms on your chart. You'll see the work zone gradually moving up in your chart, to the actions and situations that have a higher fear temperature now but that will be lower when you get to them. As you do, you'll be taking more and more of your life back from OCD.

Here are some tips for success with Step 5:

- *Take the time to learn the chill-out skills in this chapter so you'll have a backup for the brainpower skills.* Sometimes everyone needs a little more than the brainpower skills to get through the discomfort of talking back to OCD. It's important to find a way to hold out for long enough that OCD gets the message. If the fear or discomfort that comes with an obsession seems really hard to take even though you know you want to try to resist OCD, these extra techniques can get you through it.

• *Don't worry if you discover new obsessions or rituals while you're going through this program.* It doesn't mean that OCD is getting worse. It just means you've got great detective skills and are uncovering every symptom that you need to tackle to get rid of OCD. When you do discover a new symptom, be sure to add it to your hiccup and EX/RP task charts.

Get Ready

How did you do with your trial task in Step 4? Were you able to resist performing your rituals some of the time, all of the time, or not at all? You may even have done well enough to move on to another task on your list. But if you weren't entirely victorious over OCD, the purpose of reviewing Step 4 is not to beat yourself up. You're probably already an expert at beating yourself up about OCD, and that will only stand in the way of your future success. The purpose of this review is to gather information that will help you succeed in this and future steps of the program. So let's see what you found out that can help you.

First, know that it's perfectly normal during the trial tasks to feel scared, nervous, uncomfortable, antsy, or plain old bad in a way you might not be able to define. Exposing yourself to an action or situation that is tied up with OCD naturally makes you feel that way—making you feel uncomfortable is how OCD sets up that bad bargain we talked about earlier. This won't change immediately, but as you did the opposite of what OCD told you, you should have noticed those uncomfortable feelings getting milder and milder until they mostly went away. That's how EX/RP works—repeated exposure to the OCD hiccup situation without rituals eliminates the tendency to hiccup. What you need to find out today is how much discomfort you can deal with right now and how much you might be able to deal with in the days and weeks ahead.

If you were able to resist performing rituals even some of the time, you're tolerating more discomfort than you have in the past. *No matter how little you were able to resist, you've scored a victory: first, because you're doing something you weren't able to do against OCD before, but also because information is power.* What you learn from each task you do helps you figure out how to gain ground in the work zone in the next 2 weeks.

Even if you found yourself avoiding the situation or action altogether so that you weren't tempted to perform OCD's ritual, or if you went ahead and performed the ritual each time you faced the situation, you've gathered some information that makes you more powerful against OCD. You know now that *the task you chose was too hard.* All you have to do is review your symptom chart and choose a task for this week that has a lower fear temperature. Or break down the task you chose so that it'll be a bit easier. As you saw in the last chapter, there are many different ways to break a task that's too tough into smaller tasks that aren't. You might want to cut down on a ritual rather than stop it completely. You might also want to look at the fear temperature you assigned to the task you tried. Maybe it deserves a 6 instead of a 3 or a 4 after all.

Also review the strategies you used to try resisting OCD. What worked and what didn't? What did you try first, and what did you bring in as your relief pitcher? Whatever worked, keep using it, but be careful not to let OCD get you to do stuff that makes it easy in the short run but really means you're going along with OCD when you don't have to. For example, don't touch something dirty while telling yourself that you'll wash extra later. That's playing right into OCD's hands. If some tactics didn't work so well, trade them for something else or switch the order in which you use your strategies. Take a look at that brainpower card again. Did you learn anything last week that makes you think you need to rewrite your brainpower script a little?

Me and my mom went to the grocery store and I touched the meat counter, something I couldn't do before because OCD tells me that I'll get mad cow disease. This time I just laughed at him and said "No way." I still had to ask my mom whether it was OK to touch the counter, though, and I still can't touch meat, and it would have been really hard if she'd refused to answer.

—*Alex, age 12*

I don't like poopy things. I don't even like toilets. It really gets me to have to share a toilet with my stupid brother—he pees on the seat. Sometimes I have to come home from friends' homes to use the bathroom in our house. I especially don't like this part of OCD. This week I used my bathroom instead of the guest bathroom. It was hard, but I felt good about it. Really, it wasn't as bad as I thought it would be, and my brother helped out by putting the seat up.

—*Eva, age 14*

Noisy hurt my feelings this week. Noisy doesn't like chewing noises. I asked my dad to chew really loud at dinner, and it made me really upset when he wouldn't stop even when Mom told him it was too hard for me. We had a big fight, and my dad started yelling at me and my mom, and my mom ended up crying. I hate OCD, and I hate dinner so much that I'm not going to eat anymore.

—Sandra, age 6

This exercise was really helpful. I tried three ways to interrupt one of my washing rituals. One was too hard, one was too easy, and the last was just right. Interestingly enough, the one that was too hard became easy by the end of the week. This stuff really works—I was only late for the school bus because of washing once this week. I didn't have to involve my folks as they don't hang out with me in the bathroom, but I told them about it and they seemed pretty pleased.

—Sam, age 17

Every one of these kids inched forward a little into the work zone, and even Sandra and her family learned something: They now find it easier to remember that the kid with OCD makes the rules; they see that when Sandra felt her fear temperature zoom off the top of the thermometer, her dad should have listened to her and stopped chewing loudly. Together they decided he could chew so everyone could hear him, but not very loud, for about 3 minutes during dinner instead. Sandra still felt like running away from the table, but instead she asked her mom what they were going to do after school the next day and got so involved in thinking about the playground that her fear temperature dropped from the usual 3 to 1 by the time Dad had stopped chomping. By the end of the week, he could chew as much as he wanted, and they went to a movie together to celebrate.

If your fear temperature went way up during your trial tasks, you should probably break down the task to lower its temperature to begin with, as Sandra did. But if, during Step 5, you find this happening again, be sure to tell yourself that it's OK that OCD won *this time*—you'll win next time. Reassuring yourself this way will make you stronger, which is progress itself.

Before you get started on the tasks in this chapter, post the summary of Step 5 from the back of this book where you'll see it often, to remind you of what you're going to do for the next 2 weeks. Also keep your symptom chart somewhere handy. It doesn't have to be pasted up on your wall where everyone can see it if you don't want to do that, but it should be available for quick reference, with a pencil nearby for jotting notes or making any further changes that arise. You're going to collect as much data about what works and what doesn't work as you can in the next 2 weeks, so you might want to keep on hand one of the smallest size spiral notebooks for jotting down additional notes.

Get Going

Figure Out Where Family Members and Others Get Tangled Up in OCD

When your parents, brothers and sisters, teachers, friends, and others get tangled up in OCD, things usually get worse for you. Maybe your dad washes your sheets every day because OCD says they have to stay clean, and the extra work that creates for him makes you feel guilty and ashamed. Maybe your mom's frustration over OCD is getting hard for her to hide and that just makes you worry that she's not on your side anymore. Maybe your sister isn't speaking to you this week because your rituals have made the two of you late for school twice, and now she has detention. Or maybe your whole family "helps" with your rituals because they hate seeing you scared or uncomfortable—but now OCD expects you to do more rituals than ever.

There's no doubt about it: OCD can have a big impact on the people closest to you. If your family or friends get involved in rituals, the fight against OCD isn't just your fight. A little later in the program you can decide whether and how you want to recruit your family and others in resisting OCD. But first you have to figure out any ways other people get tangled up in OCD. Ask yourself: How does OCD boss around your parents, your siblings, or anyone else besides you? What do you think the fear temperature would be for you if they bossed OCD back? See if you can add these actions, situations, or triggers and their fear temperatures to your symptom chart.

> *My mom serves me special food. She doesn't like it, but I won't eat any-thing that she doesn't make the way OCD tells me 'cause I might get sick.*
> —*Christina, age 8*

> *I make (actually OCD makes—sorry) my sister wash her hands before she uses the TV remote. She gets really ticked at me, but I can't help it, and it makes me mad when my parents yell at me because she and I fight all the time. All this yelling makes it harder for me to resist.*
> —*Kurt, age 17*

I have to ask my teacher if I cheated. She knows I have OCD, so she just tells me no, but sometimes I have to ask her a bunch of times, and I can tell she doesn't like it when I waste her time. Sometimes instead of asking, I'll just put down the wrong answer, but then everyone thinks I'm stupid or I haven't studied. I sure wish everyone understood what it was like to have OCD.

—Alice, age 12

Choose New Symptoms to Work On—with a Little Help from Your EX/RP Trial Task

Here's where you'll see how useful the information you gathered last week can be. Pull out your symptom chart so you can choose a new target or two for this week and next. If you had a hard time with your trial task, pick a symptom with a lower fear temperature. If you found the task amazingly easy, consider tackling one with the same fear temperature or one a little higher up the ladder.

Here are a couple of things to take into account when choosing tasks for the next 2 weeks:

• Think of each task as either a situation you create or one that happens naturally. In other words, there are actions or situations or triggers that you can avoid (and usually do when controlled by OCD), as well as ones you can't avoid. You're going to want to tackle both kinds, maybe one of each for Step 5.

Created Tasks

For these tasks you purposely put yourself in contact with something that you could normally avoid. For example, if OCD makes you worry about getting contaminated by a certain doorknob in your house, and ordinarily you just don't use that door, for your task you would seek out that doorknob, touch it, and then not wash your hands. In this case avoiding the doorknob is a kind of ritual you perform to control the bad feelings caused by the obsession. So the EX part of the task involves not only not avoiding the doorknob but seeking it out and touching it on purpose.

Natural Tasks

These are the situations or actions you can't avoid, so your only choice for the task is to focus on resisting performing a ritual. Let's say you have a ritual related to choosing clothes to wear to school. Unless you want to go to school without clothes on (and you have to go to school), OCD has you over a barrel. Ordinarily, while under the control of OCD, you would perform a ritual. But now you know that you can stop, interrupt, or change the ritual so that you don't have to do what OCD says.

- You need to know what kind of resistance you put up before you can judge how well you did with your trial task and whether you need to try something easier or harder this week. Successfully resisting OCD in the first category means staying in contact with the trigger, resisting the urge to leave. Successfully resisting OCD in the second category means staying in contact with the trigger without performing your usual ritual; it does *not* mean resisting the urge to perform the ritual by bailing out early. You need to stay with the task until your fear thermometer comes down to a 1 or 2 and stays there. And then wait a little longer. Otherwise, OCD wins, and it'll be as hard or harder to do this task the next time. **If you start a task, finish it.** If you don't feel that you can go all the way to the end, then do the best you can without starting an intentional EX/RP task. Some days are tough, and it is OK if you just don't have it in you not to be hard on yourself. But most of the time you need to start the EX/RP homework and complete it successfully day after day until OCD is no more. There's nothing more important.

You also need to make sure you haven't just traded one ritual for another. Sometimes kids avoid performing a ritual by telling themselves something like "If I do the ritual, something bad will happen." In this case they haven't actually taken back any territory from OCD, because they feel just as scared or squirmy at the end of the task as they did at the beginning. They haven't performed the usual ritual, but they've played OCD's game by going through a mental ritual—making doing the ritual "illegal," with the same bad bargain from OCD: if they do perform the ritual, they'll feel bad. Delaying a ritual such as washing until later when no one will notice is another good example of how OCD can trick you into doing its business.

In general, it's still important to pick a symptom that you can already resist pretty well. Proceeding too fast into OCD's territory will only set you back and rob you of valuable time and confidence. Look at your symptom chart and see which hiccups in your work zone you could target as created tasks and which as natural tasks. Which do you feel more comfortable targeting right now? Here's another area in which you have control. If you think it will be easier to resist if you purposely expose yourself to something that will bring on your obsessions and then resist running away, choose one of those to tackle first. If you feel more confident trying to avoid performing your rituals when you run into a situation you usually can't avoid, choose one of those.

Once you've picked one or two more tasks to try, start practicing them as "homework" for 30 to 60 minutes per day. Pay careful attention (with your parents' help, if necessary) to the fear thermometer during the tasks. Remember, your goal is to get the temperature down to 0 or 1. There's lots of extra help in this chapter to keep you from bailing out on the task, which is really important to make sure you keep shrinking OCD's territory. Once you've been able to do a task without the fear thermometer going over a 0 or 1 *for 2 to 3 days in a row*, you've moved that symptom (or that portion of a symptom) out of the work zone and into your territory.

Congratulations! When this happens, cross it off your task list and your symptom chart and keep moving up the ladder of that task list. Pick another task to target, and keep going. Do the same thing each time you've been able to do a task without any discomfort for 2 to 3 days in a row.

For teenagers: Do the work on your own; you know your own mind. If appropriate, let your parents review your choices. Certainly if they're involved in the rituals or trigger the obsessions, you'll have to involve them in the process of choosing EX/RP targets. Your trial task may have made you feel pretty confident in your abilities, and you *should* feel confident. That doesn't mean, however, that you should make things harder for yourself during the next 2 weeks. If your parents suggest that you may have chosen a task that's too hard, try to believe that this is not one of those times when they're trying to hold you back and treat you like a child. If you haven't already had some success resisting OCD with the task you've picked, you're setting yourself up for failure, which will only cost you time.

Another potential stumbling block is that you've amassed quite a collection of rules, morals, and traditions by the time you've reached adolescence, and it can be hard to disentangle those from your obsessions. If you're having violent thoughts, for example, your moral code may tell you it's wrong to allow such thoughts into your head. Shame over these thoughts may keep you from treating them like any other OCD trigger, which may mean you won't have the chance to conquer them. Or what if you find yourself repelled by thoughts about promiscuity or sexual orientation? Are those ideas coming from the culture in which you live, from your religious beliefs, or from OCD? If you have any doubts at all, or if you end up confused about what should be on your symptom chart in the first place, talk to someone. Your parents are one possibility; a therapist is another. For kids with religious OCD, talking with a priest or minister can be helpful, but as with parents and therapists, be sure to find one who knows about OCD.

Resisting Obsessions and Mental Rituals

If you need extra help dealing with obsessions or if your rituals are mainly mental ones, here are a couple of good ways to learn to beat OCD on this ground. You can try both, or see if one appeals to you more than the other and concentrate on that:

1. *Establish a "worry time."* Let's say OCD has you worrying that you might have sinned by thinking something normal, such as getting mad at your sister for something she did. To cancel out this thought, OCD makes you say some specific prayers and tells you that if you don't you and your sister both will go to hell. These praying rituals tend to go on all day, off and on, no matter when the ritual was first triggered. You know your sister will trigger the obsession—that's a given—so just do your best to resist performing the praying ritual. Also, assign two 10- to 20-minute periods, say one in the morning and one in the afternoon, as "worry time," during which you purposely invite your obsession into your head but don't do the praying ritual. During the assigned time, not only let the obsession enter your mind but also purposely repeat it over and over as though it were true: "I'm going to hell for being mad at my sister and so is she." *Don't* use positive thoughts or other diversions to avoid getting anxious. The idea is to intentionally make yourself as distressed over the obsession as possible. Keep this up until the discomfort wanes to a 1 or 2 on the fear thermometer. If you're having trouble with an obsession or praying ritual at other times, tell yourself you can resist it now, because you're going to defer it till the next worry time. Lots of kids find this helps them succeed in beating OCD outside their dedicated worry times.

2. *Make a tape of the obsessive thought or mental ritual and listen to it over and over.* At a time when the obsession comes up, write down what you're thinking, word for word. Then, at another time, record yourself on a tape or digital voice recorder while reading the thoughts back to yourself, using the tone of voice that reflects how you feel while the obsession is taking hold. Or you can simply turn the recorder on and make your recording during a time when an obsession is taking hold and skip the writing step. Then, once a day, schedule 30 to 45 minutes during which you'll listen to the tape over and over, using headphones, to make yourself feel as distressed as you can, just to show OCD that you can do it. Don't do the ritual that goes with the obsession, however, or the exercise will not work.

Most kids who try these techniques to trick OCD start out feeling pretty bad during worry time or while listening to their tapes. But toward the end of the time period they're starting to get pretty bored with the whole thing. I'd be willing to bet that by the end of the week you won't even be able to get yourself upset over the obsession during these practice times. That's exactly what you want: You've gotten so used to this particular idea that it doesn't bother you anymore. Score 1 for you, 0 for OCD.

Learn to Break OCD's Rules

Here's where the real fun begins. So far you've been making trial runs into enemy territory, a scary but, I hope, ultimately reassuring exercise to show you that you *can* take charge and you *can* take back control of your life. Maybe what you've accomplished is standing your ground or forging ahead instead of taking an escape route when you know something that triggers an obsession is on the horizon. If OCD tends to send you on a maze-like route to avoid the things that bother you, that can be quite an accomplishment. But now you're going to take your resistance a little further. It's time to refine your ability to resist rituals.

Rituals are whatever OCD says you have to do if you want to stop feeling bad when an obsession comes up. They are the "rules" set by OCD that you need to learn to break. They aren't your rules; they belong to OCD. Don't let anyone tell you differently. Your trial task should have shown you that breaking OCD's rules does not have to be as frightening as OCD has threatened in the past. But it's only natural to feel a little nervous about breaking OCD's rules, so let me set your mind at rest about this with three ideas: (1) You have a variety of options for breaking the rules, which will allow you to do this gradually; (2) you can have some fun here, because this part of Step 5 gives you an opportunity to use your imagination to the max; (3) nothing bad will happen if you don't do what OCD tells you to do, but you will get rid of OCD.

Four Ways to Break OCD's Rules

OCD is greedy. It likes its power over you so much that it would love to have more. And if it can't have more, then it wants things to be done exactly the same way all the time. If Germy makes you wash your hands 15 times after every ride in a "dirty" car, then Germy will be happiest if you start washing your hands 20 times or if you start washing your hands every time you go a friend's house, too. Although Germy will settle for your simply following the original rules religiously, it'll try to expand into new places if you let it. So don't let it, especially now that you're doing your best to resist OCD in an organized way.

From your experience in the preceding weeks, you now know not only that can you break Germy's rules without paying a huge fine but also that you stand only to gain if you do break those rules. So I'm going to give you four ways to make breaking OCD's rules a way of life. (Just don't extend this approach to rules set by Mom and Dad or your teachers.) These ways of pulling a switch on OCD are similar to what you may already have done in setting up a hiccup ladder for a single symptom that's giving you a really hard time.

1. *Delay the ritual.* If Germy says you have to wash your hands right after riding in a car or using the toilet, break this rule by waiting for a preplanned period of time before you wash. Try 10 or 15 minutes—whatever you think you can do—and if that works, gradually work your way up to 30 minutes, then an hour, and so forth until you've waited Germy out and he's gone home in a sulk. Eventually, you'll need to stop washing altogether to prove the point to OCD (then you can start normal washing again), but you may or may not be there yet.

2. *Shorten the ritual.* Germy says you have to wash your hands 15 times after a car ride? Try 10 times for a couple of days. Then reduce it to 5 times, and keep cutting back until you don't need to wash at all. You can do this with time (wash for 5 minutes by the clock and then quit, whether you feel like it or not) or by reducing the number of repetitions. Same thing for other kinds of rituals. Pray for a shorter period of time or say fewer prayers. Arrange less, check less, count less, and so on. Set up what you'll do in advance and then stick to it.

3. *Do the ritual differently.* If Germy says you have to use the bathroom closest to the front door to wash your hands, use the upstairs bathroom instead. If he says you have to wash your left hand first and then your right, switch on him. Here's where you can get creative. Get the ritual out of order, put something in the middle of the ritual that doesn't belong there—singing a part of a song is a good one—or do only a part of the ritual. However you change the ritual, make sure you do it *your* way.

4. *Do the ritual slowly.* Maybe you're used to rushing through your 15 hand washings to get the ritual over with. You know, though, that that doesn't make it any easier or less disturbing to you. You also know it doesn't do anything to get Germy off your back. Try slowing things down. Instead of quickly going through the 15 hand washings, wash your hands really slowly, say twice. Don't let OCD run away with your mind, but pay attention to what is really happening. For example, take a lot of care and pay attention to the details—the way the slippery soap feels between your fingers, its scent, the squeaky feeling once you've rinsed, and so forth. Or let's say OCD makes you spend an hour checking whether the lamp plug is pulled out of its socket. If asked, you might say that you're checking to be sure it is out, but what is really happening is that you are thinking obsessively about the house burning down and funerals and so on. Try one repetition of the ritual in which you put the plug in the socket, paying careful attention to the intention to move your hand, the feeling of moving, the resistance when it hits the socket, the intention to push a little harder, the actual movement until the plug stops. Then reverse the process, watching the intention to back the plug out before you watch the actual movement. When the plug is out (you know this because you're watching what happens, not thinking thoughts of doom), set it down, say "OUT," and walk away. This technique is very helpful for mindless repeating rituals of all sorts, but particularly checking and grooming rituals. Before you know it, what was once a mindless ritual is a whole different experience—one in which you're in charge.

Over the next 2 weeks, get as creative as you can in breaking the rules. Channel all the energy that you might ordinarily put into trying to stay up just a few more minutes past bedtime or getting just a little more videogame time or avoiding chores for just a little longer into breaking OCD's rules. Your parents will thank you. You'll thank yourself. OCD will not thank you. But it won't be able to do a thing about it.

Breaking the rules this way is a great alternative to trying to resist performing a ritual altogether. Sometimes that's just too hard, and pushing yourself to go "cold turkey" will only make you feel that you've failed. Learn to break the rules, and before you know it you've moved another symptom from OCD's territory into yours.

For teenagers: Many people believe that if they don't perform rituals the anxiety will overwhelm them and they'll go crazy, so if you're finding it hard to resist performing rituals for the obsession you've targeted this week, don't label yourself "weak" or "wimpy." Just try a little irreverence and break some rules. This might be one of the most valuable tools to add to your kit. We know you're creative, so use it here. Remember what my friend and colleague Lee Baer (see his book in the Resources) says to his patients when they ask how they can possibly resist such strong compulsions: "Any way you can."

Become a Scientist Yourself

A lot of very smart scientists working with kids like you have worked hard on creating this program. Scientists are curious about why things work and why they don't work. They are always interested in what's actually happening and don't like to be fooled. Scientists conduct experiments to be sure that their theories are correct. This sounds like you, doesn't it? You're investigating OCD so you know how it works and conducting your own experiments with your symptoms to prove that OCD is just nonsense so your brain will know it can stop hiccupping.

To move forward, constantly (if slowly) increasing the size of your territory and shrinking OCD's territory, you need to be sure that the temperature on your fear thermometer is going down for the task you've chosen to work on during these 2 weeks. If it's not, you'll want to find out what's going wrong as soon as possible so that you don't get discouraged and lose ground. Think of your resistance efforts as a scientific experiment. If you can't reduce the fear that you feel when some-

Chill-Out Skills

To see OCD clearly, you first have to relax, then observe and accept that OCD is present while you let it pass. If you get so tense during your chosen tasks and your brainpower skills just aren't enough, try learning one of these ways to relax your body, which will help your mind relax, too.

Deep Breathing

Following your breath is a great way to anchor your body in the present so you don't get lost in OCD or, if you do get lost, to bring you back into the present, where you can deal with OCD skillfully. Have you ever watched a basketball player at the foul line? Maybe you noticed how many of them pause and slowly blow air in and out of their mouths before shooting. The reason is that when you're tense, you don't make very good foul shots—and you don't talk back to OCD very well. When you're tense, you breathe so much from your chest that you may even feel as though you can't catch your breath, which only makes you tenser. Learning deep breathing will help you relax so you can concentrate on resisting OCD (or making a great free throw): Start by lying down on your back. Put a light pillow or something like it on your stomach. If you're feeling tense right now, notice how the pillow doesn't move even though you're breathing. Now take a breath and say out loud, "Ha, ha, ha." See how the pillow moves? That's because you're now breathing from your diaphragm, which is the way we should all breathe, all the time. To learn better how to do this, take a deep, slow breath in through your nose, inhaling as much air as you can. Did the pillow rise? Good! Now hold your breath for a count of 3 and then exhale as slowly as you can, watching the pillow go back down. Practice this about 10 times until you feel like you've got it. Now try the next skill.

Relaxation

This is an old trick, and it works. You might want to get a parent or therapist to help you learn this, but basically here's how it works: Sit or lie down somewhere that's comfortable. Take some deep breaths that make your stomach stick way out and then flatten when you exhale. Now count to 5 or 10 while you tighten up your neck muscles by shrugging your shoulders. Then slowly relax your neck muscles while you count back from 10 or 5 to 1. Now drop your head forward so your chin touches your chest, slowly drop your head to one side, then to your back, then to the other side, and back forward again. Repeat. Now lift your arms with your palms up to a count of 5 or 10 and then lower them, counting back to 1. Do the same thing with the rest of your body, tensing and then relaxing your hands, stomach, legs, and finally feet. If you want you can repeat the whole exercise from your feet back to your neck. End with more deep breathing. I bet you feel really relaxed now. If you practice this routine every day for a while, you'll be able to start the drill during a task that you find just too uncomfortable to finish.

OK, now here's the short form to use whenever you need it to keep from getting lost in OCD: First, take a deep breath and let it out slowly to anchor yourself in your body. Look around and see what's happening. OK, now that you know where you are, let your body relax. Breathe. Accept that OCD is present, but don't go on and on in your mind about it. Rather, do the best you can in that moment to skillfully resist OCD.

thing triggers an obsession or if you can't begin to resist performing rituals, you need to look at each step of the "experiment" and see what's going wrong. Here are some possibilities to consider:

- *Are you substituting a new ritual for an old one?* We mentioned earlier how common this is. The boy who felt compelled by OCD to wash his hands 15 times after every car ride started telling himself that the car really wasn't full of germs and that his hands were perfectly clean when he got out. On the way into the house, he'd hold his hands out in front of him, look at them, turn them over and look at the other side, and tell himself that they definitely looked clean. By the fifth time he had done this, he found himself turning his hands over and over as he looked at them on the way into the house. He wasn't washing his hands anymore, so he couldn't understand why his anxiety was still so high. It turns out that he had substituted a new ritual—turning his hands over repeatedly to check for any signs of "contamination"—for the hand washing. Same obsession, different ritual, same old anxiety.

- *Are you giving up on a task too soon?* Most of the time the fear thermometer registers a drop after you stick it out for 20-30 minutes. But not always. Sometimes it takes up to an hour. If your fear temperature isn't dropping on this task, try extending the task a little. If the temperature does go down then, you'll have to make your task practices a little longer for a while until you can get it down to 1 or 2 each time. Zero is even better. If this feels pretty tough, remember: When you bail out on a task before OCD gives up, OCD feels like it's won and will come back with more confidence instead of less. Hang in there!

- *Have you picked a task that's too hard?* If you're not substituting a mental ritual, and you're not abandoning the task too early, then you have to consider the possibility that you need to pick a task that has a lower rating from your symptom chart. Remember, you gain nothing by making success impossible to achieve.

Good scientists are diligent and objective. They look squarely at the facts and never make up test results. So don't kid yourself. Use unwavering scrutiny to report on your own experiments with OCD. Don't let OCD obscure your vision. Your abilities as a scientist will keep you going through this program until you've won back most of your territory from OCD. For example, when you take note of which rule-breaking method(s) and which tool(s) from your kit seem to help you most, you can make those your first choices when you have to face OCD on a new battlefront.

How a therapist can help: If you can't figure out why your fear temperature isn't going down or why it suddenly dropped altogether for a certain task, your therapist is the best source of help.

Taking Stock

Fill out the OCD scale once more and, again, plot your numbers on your graph. Take a look at your "Getting Stronger Every Day" form. Did you manage to do your practice tasks for 30-60 minutes every day?

Even better, take a look at your symptom chart and task lists. You should be starting to see that you're working your way up the ladder, resisting at harder and harder tasks, expanding your territory and shrinking OCD's. Keep up the great work!

At the end of each day, check off whether you've followed the instructions for the step, spending 30–60 minutes a day. Some kids don't feel like they need a full 3 weeks for Step 5. If you end up moving on to Step 6 after 2 weeks, check off that homework too as you complete it. **But don't feel like you've blown it if you don't add in Step 6 during these 3 weeks.**

Day 15 ☐ I did the homework for Step 5.

Day 16 ☐ I did the homework for Step 5.

Day 17 ☐ I did the homework for Step 5.

Day 18 ☐ I did the homework for Step 5.

Day 19 ☐ I did the homework for Step 5.

Day 20 ☐ I did the homework for Step 5.

Day 21 ☐ I did the homework for Step 5.

Day 22 ☐ I did the homework for Step 5.

Day 23 ☐ I did the homework for Step 5.

Day 24 ☐ I did the homework for Step 5.

Day 25 ☐ I did the homework for Step 5.

Day 26 ☐ I did the homework for Step 5.

Day 27 ☐ I did the homework for Step 5.

Day 28 ☐ I did the homework for Step 5.

Day 29 ☐ I did the homework for Step 5.   ☐ I did the homework for Step 6.

Day 30 ☐ I did the homework for Step 5.   ☐ I did the homework for Step 6.

Day 31 ☐ I did the homework for Step 5.   ☐ I did the homework for Step 6.

Day 32 ☐ I did the homework for Step 5.   ☐ I did the homework for Step 6.

Day 33 ☐ I did the homework for Step 5.   ☐ I did the homework for Step 6.

Day 34 ☐ I did the homework for Step 5.   ☐ I did the homework for Step 6.

Day 35 ☐ I did the homework for Step 5.   ☐ I did the homework for Step 6.

Step 5: Instructions for Parents

THERE'S A LOT TO GET DONE at this step, and your child's work gets more complicated. Naturally, this calls for lots of support from you. But it also may mean you'll have to assist with some of the work involving new skills. If you do, remember to defer to your child in any way you can. *Ask* if you can help with something that you know your child has to learn at this step. This will notify your child that you know what the program entails and that you intend to stay on top of it without nagging him to get things done on your schedule. Here are a couple of tips for success at this step:

- *Avoid indiscriminate praise.* As your child dives into exposure and response prevention (EX/RP) tasks, your main task—support—also gets more complicated. In your role as a cheerleader, it may be hard to know when to praise your child. Sure, it's important to be positive about your child's efforts, especially if OCD has created a generally negative atmosphere defined by frustration and anger and guilt in your home. But now you need to be sure that you don't praise your child indiscriminately in the name of increasing her self-esteem. So much has been made of the importance of self-esteem that many of us have forgotten what instills it. Empty praise never raises a child's self-esteem; accomplishment does. So reserve your praise for your child's real accomplishments. Kids with OCD have enough anxiety to deal with. They don't need to add performance anxiety, which is exactly what develops when parents toss meaningless compliments their way in an effort to make a child feel good. Being praised for nothing backfires, instilling fear that the child will never measure up when she really does try hard at an exposure task. So it's best not only to limit praise to concrete accomplishments but, as suggested in Chapter 5, to put the praise in terms of how *your child* is likely to feel about his victories, not how *you* feel.
- *Don't push your child to resist OCD too fast.* When you start to see your child succeed with EX/RP tasks, it's easy to become impatient and want him to step up the

199

When you praise your child for victories over OCD:

Say "You must feel really good about resisting OCD in the bathroom for 2 days in a row!"

Instead of "I'm so proud of what you've been doing recently!"

Say "You should give yourself a big pat on the back for sticking with your OCD homework on a day when you had all that school homework, too."

Instead of "You always work so hard—good job!"

When your child is disappointed in being unable to resist a certain ritual:

Say "Why don't you go look at that chart and see how much you've accomplished already."

Instead of "You're doing great!"

When your child hasn't done all the homework:

Say "I heard you scored a goal today" or "That sculpture you did in art class looks like it must have taken a lot of work."

Instead of "You're terrific" or "Keep up the good work with OCD!" Focusing on other specific, positive achievements and ignoring the fact that the homework hasn't been completed is probably the best move, at least as long as it's just a brief lapse. If your child continues to avoid the homework, try to feel him out about his commitment to the program or talk to your child's therapist.

5

pace and get rid of OCD once and for all. After all, if he can do it with this one situation, he can do it everywhere, right? Wrong. If your child's OCD symptoms have been causing great inconvenience for your family, or if the child's grades have been falling or you and your child's other parent have gotten mired in conflict over the illness, your child already knows that you want OCD gone as fast as possible. In many kids with OCD this awareness is enough to cause debilitating anxiety that you'll push too hard and expect too much. Your child absolutely must feel it's OK to risk failure, or he won't put the necessary effort into the EX/RP tasks, much less succeed at them.

If you find yourself feeling overly optimistic about your child's first trial task, pick up that symptom chart and look right at the circled work zone—those are the *only* symptoms that your child should consider targeting for exposure and response prevention right now. In fact, it wouldn't hurt to anticipate your child's worry that you'll be impatient and reinforce your understanding of the work zone by saying things like "You're doing a really good job of sticking to the work zone, honey. That's exactly what you should be doing during this step."

Get Ready

Help your child review the trial task from Step 4 unless she's a teenager or otherwise quite independent. Now is the time for the child to learn how to make an accurate assessment of his success with a task, because knowing where things went right or wrong is critical to picking the next task for the work zone.

Get Going

Figure Out Where Family Members and Others Get Tangled Up in OCD

You'll need to participate in this part of Step 5, because it may be hard for your child to untangle your role in OCD on her own. Or you may be one of the lucky families who are not involved in doing OCD's rituals. (In that case, read the following, but you don't need to put it into play.) Some of the ways you're entangled in OCD will be obvious. If you agree to do much more cleaning than you would ordinarily do, or if you change the family's routine in any other concrete way, the fact that you're entangled will be inescapable. But there are other ways to be bossed around by OCD that may not be as blatant.

Sometimes, meeting OCD's demands masquerades as normal family interactions. OCD told one girl we know that her mother would not be wearing enough clothing to stay warm during the day, and because of this something bad would happen to her, so she would ask her mother for the weather report every morning. Telling her daughter what it would be like outside so the daughter could talk with her mother about how to dress appears on the surface to be a perfectly normal thing to do. But in this case, the routine was part of OCD's territory because it was a way of unknowingly yielding to the daughter's obsession by performing a reassurance ritual.

OCD told another little girl that if she didn't eat the foods at her meals in a certain order, in carefully measured amounts, she would get sick. So she would ask her mother what the family was having for dinner that night right after she got home from school. Again, this is not an unusual question for a child to ask, nor an unusual type of information for a parent to supply. But in this case OCD was pulling the strings. The mother *had* to plan meals far enough ahead so that she could report accurately at 3:00 what they would be eating, and even though the meals seemed to be what any average American family might eat, the mother had been combining the "right" types of foods in each dinner for so long that she no longer realized she was acceding to OCD's demands.

Being asked to focus on how you're trapped in OCD may make you uncomfortable. You might feel guilty at the suggestion that you could have been "causing" your child to have OCD or "making it worse." Be assured that you're not to blame.

But it's important to know how you're involved, because OCD is likely wreaking some degree of havoc with your whole family's social and community relationships and may be having a deleterious effect on your relationship with your child as well. Just having to go to the doctor or even doing this program is one sign of how OCD affects your family. Understanding your involvement in the illness is the first step toward extricating yourself so that you too can make OCD the problem and turn your attention to being as supportive as possible of your child's efforts to show OCD the door. So try not to hold back. Look honestly and tenderly at any of your behaviors that might be influenced by OCD and at how you respond to your child's discomfort when OCD arises and to the resulting need to perform rituals.

Reassurance seeking is part of OCD rituals for many kids. Sometimes it's an overt part of a ritual, but sometimes it's hard to connect to OCD. Sometimes it's normal, not OCD at all. When a child has an obsession involving worry that the doors and windows aren't all locked at night and that therefore someone will get in, asking for your reassurance that the doors and windows *are* locked is an overt way of using reassurance seeking as an anxiety-calming ritual. Once is OK, twice is marginal, and more than that is not healthy. But what about the child who gives you a seemingly innocent morning hug but is really doing so because OCD is getting him to check to be sure that his bad thought didn't cause you to get cancer? Would you be aware that the child is asking for reassurance that a future consequence has been averted and therefore engaging in avoidance and subverting her efforts to resist OCD?

Helping younger kids: The younger the child, the more dependent he or she will be on parental assistance. A child who still needs Mom or Dad to help him dress in the morning, complete a bedtime routine, make social plans, and get everywhere he needs to go will likely involve parents in many if not all of his responses to the obsessions that OCD imposes on him—so much so, in fact, that the child and the parents may have gotten to the point where a lot of their OCD-dictated behavior just seems like business as usual. This means that you will be indispensable in ferreting out the ways that you and other family members are involved in OCD.

Helping teenagers: This can be a tough nut to crack, as teenagers are supposed to be trying to become more, not less, independent, as often happens when OCD involves parents and siblings in rituals. Not surprisingly, when OCD gets in the way of a teen's desire to be her own boss, it can spark conflicts even when it is clear that the teen's parent is in the right and only trying to be helpful. For example, it's not uncommon for a teen with grooming rituals to get trapped in the bathroom and need help to get unstuck so as to make it to school on time. However, that help isn't always welcome and isn't always offered in the most constructive way, which leaves everyone feeling sad, mad, and at a loss about what to do. So, what to do? Try to set conflict aside and map in some detail what actually happens so that you'll know how to address it using EX/RP and the other tools learned in this program.

Serena, age 16, had a long, intricate series of rituals that had to be done in order every morning before she could go to school. Because the family had

---

What If You, Too, Have OCD or Have Some Other Kind of Mental Illness?

Twenty percent of the children who have OCD have a parent or sibling who also has OCD. Many of the rest have a parent with anxiety or depression. If you have OCD yourself, you may find yourself getting involved in your child's obsessions and compulsions, whether or not you have the same sorts of obsessions and compulsions. The worst situation, of course, is to have the same kind of OCD and get trapped together in rituals. Another problem comes when someone in the family has a different kind of mental illness—not OCD—that interacts with OCD. For example, it's very hard for a depressed parent to do what's necessary to help a child resist OCD. A sibling with ADHD who takes a lot of effort to keep on track may make it very difficult for a parent to devote attention to helping resist OCD. If you find it hard to consider extricating yourself from OCD's territory because of OCD or another form of mental illness, you will need to seek the help of a therapist or physician who can help you address your own mental health needs.

---

three kids, two parents, and only two bathrooms, OCD was causing problems for everyone. Serena's brother, Angelo, was always pounding on the bathroom door trying to hurry Serena up. Serena's dad would sometimes do the same. Poor Serena would get so frustrated she'd yell "shut up," knowing full well that it meant she had to start over. Once they all understood what was happening—that interrupting the ritual made it longer—Serena got a dedicated bathroom for 3 months while she diligently worked on getting rid of OCD. After a while, OCD in the bathroom shrank enough to make room for Angelo. He took Serena to a movie with some friends, the first time they'd had fun together in a long time.

Your teenager should take the lead on this, as she usually knows better than you do what's working and what's not, but sometimes you will be better able to organize the information. Talk it over with your teenager, as much as possible like equals trying to solve a problem collaboratively.

How a therapist can help: OCD is a tricky creature that can spin a very complicated web. Sometimes other factors, such as a lot of arguing that has nothing to do with OCD, get in the way of focusing on the treatment of OCD. If you can't figure out how to ally against OCD or decode how OCD traps family members in rituals, you'll be better off asking for the help of a therapist experienced in disentangling families from OCD.

Choose New Symptoms to Work On—with a Little Help from Your Child's Trial Task

While your child is choosing a series of rituals to resist for the next 2 weeks, think about what kinds of diversions you can use to help the child pass the time while refraining from doing rituals. Are there word games you both like to play? Can you get the child involved in planning dinner? Can you initiate a review of the child's schedule for the next day? Ask about homework? What can *you* do to resist the urge to give advice or to get entangled in OCD as you watch your child struggling with the emotional discomfort that the exposure task causes?

Helping younger kids: If your child is very young, you'll be involved all the way in this part of Step 5. Your child will need to be led through the entire process of reviewing the symptom chart, looking at the fear thermometer to identify the work zone, and choosing a series of EX/RP targets for the 2 weeks ahead. To do this effectively, you have to ask the right questions, help your child stick to the plan, and remain encouraging and patient so that you can elicit information and decisions from your child without simply doing the work yourself.

You may be tempted, as all parents are numerous times during the day, to rush things along, making a choice yourself just to get it done. Do whatever you can to resist this urge. Your child absolutely needs to make the choice of tasks from the work zone if he is to have a good chance of success in fighting them. If the child draws a blank when reviewing the symptom chart, read out the symptoms that are currently in the work zone rather than picking one to suggest. Think about how ritual prevention can be modified so that the EX/RP task will generate manageable discomfort. Stimulate thought and elicit responses; don't manipulate your child into choosing the task you think is best—even if the symptom is one that causes you great inconvenience and that you'd like to be rid of as soon as possible.

How a therapist can help: A therapist may be particularly helpful if your child and you are having trouble sorting out OCD symptoms from the ordinary rules of daily living. It's hard not to wash your hands after using the toilet when that's your custom, but you may have to model not washing when your child is confronting OCD. It's best to agree that this is part of treatment for OCD and not a family rule. Teens sometimes have identity issues that get tangled up with OCD. Because these often involve the need to separate from the family (simply put, to grow up and become more independent), a therapist can often be more helpful than a parent in sorting out these issues from OCD. As always, if OCD or your family situation is too complicated to manage this program on your own, it is better to get help than to flounder along alone.

Learn to Break OCD's Rules

Learning to break OCD's rules gives you a valuable opportunity to establish solidarity with your child against OCD. Ordinarily, you make the rules, and you enforce them, too. Kids know you're really on their side when suddenly you start encouraging them to break rules. So make it as fun and as wildly creative as possible. "Germy says you have to be in that bathroom washing your hands for 20 minutes, eh?" you might say to your son. "Well, how does 2 minutes sound? Take that, Germy! *We* make the rules around here." Or how about "Soap? Who says you have to wash with *soap*? How about ketchup? No, wait . . . how about salad dressing . . . or chocolate milk?" Getting goofy about rule breaking not only plants you firmly on your child's side but also calls into play the humor that should be right at the top of your child's toolkit.

Helping younger kids: Fun is even more important here, but you may have to set the tone. Younger kids will need a lot of coaching to get them on a creative roll.

How a therapist can help: This is an important step in the program, so if you're having trouble making any headway, a therapist will set up an EX/RP task for you in his or her office so that you can practice in an environment that feels more secure. This might be done in imagination or at the office, or the therapist could come to your home or go to school with your child to support him in completing an exposure successfully. Sometimes all it takes is a professional helper your child trusts to get him over the hump, and then he'll be on his way.

Become a Scientist Yourself

Keep up cheerleading, but also gently ask your child how things are going, and be specific. If your child reports blithely that going somewhere in the car never even makes her feel scared anymore, don't assume that she's conquered this obsession overnight. Total failure of an action or situation to cause anxiety is sometimes a sign that a child has substituted a new ritual, mental or behavioral. You want to help your child become aware of being sidetracked in these ways so that you can nudge her back on course if she needs it. On the other hand, success is success, and well-placed praise and, if appropriate, a thank-you is usually appreciated.

Helping younger kids: You may have to do most of the scientific observation and any recording that seems like a good idea. Young kids don't make particularly scrupulous scientists!

Taking Stock

Encourage your child to look at the symptom chart and task list with you so you can both see how different things are now than they were a few short weeks ago. Pat yourself on the back while you're patting your child on the back. And get ready for more work . . . your child is really making headway now. If not, get a therapist's help.

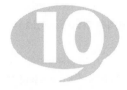

Step 6: I'm in Charge Now

BELIEVE IT OR NOT, you're a veteran now. Instead of running away, you've been out there taking on OCD on purpose and winning more and more of your life back. The work you are doing is good for your life and good for your brain, which is learning how to turn off OCD on its own. Take a moment and look at how far you've come. A long way, but not quite far enough. Now you're going to give it everything you've got. If you don't feel quite like a veteran now, you will by the end of Step 6. You've proven you can beat OCD in more places than you ever thought possible. Take advantage of the confidence you've gained and keep working away at your symptom list. It's only a matter of time before OCD drops away and you have your whole life back again.

The Game Plan for Step 6

After reviewing what you accomplished in Step 5, follow the directions under "Get Ready." Then you're going to spend 4 to 6 weeks on the instructions for Step 6, though you'll probably end up starting on Step 7 during the same time period. This is your first of two big runs talking back to OCD. You'll be working your way up the task list, relentlessly chipping away at OCD and taking control of your life back.

You're about to enter the intermediate stage of the program. You're no longer just testing your strength; now you'll be putting it to full use. You won't be trying just one task at a time to see how it goes and figure out where the chinks are in OCD's armor. Now you're going to add EX/RP tasks, doing them over and over until you repeatedly do so well in that situation that you can cross that OCD hiccup off on your chart. This means doing 30 to 60 minutes of exposure (whether natural or created, all at once or strung out like beads on a chain) and then not doing rituals for however long it takes, every day, 7 days a week. It is no accident that we call the place where you select EX/RP tasks the *work zone*. It is a big-time serious effort, but think about how good it will feel not to have OCD waiting around every corner. Your life needs this, and your brain absolutely needs it. There really is nothing more important than getting well again. Every symptom you cross off expands your territory and shrinks OCD's. Step 6 is where you really start to feel in charge. In recognition of your advances against OCD, you're going to make celebrating your success a big part of the program.

After 4 weeks, take stock. If all went well, you'll start bringing your parents (or brothers and sisters) into the action a little more closely than you may already have been doing, with their agreement and help in ending their cooperation with OCD.

As usual, put up your "Getting Stronger Every Day" chart where you'll see it before you go to bed and check off completion of your tasks for the day.

Get Ready

For the last 2 or 3 weeks you've been using your toolkit to break the rules set by OCD for hiccups down near the low end of your task list. If by the end of the second week you were able to keep your fear temperature at a 1 or even a 0 for these hiccups in the work zone for 2 or 3 days in a row, you've won this territory back from OCD. Congratulations! You can now cross these items off on your symptom chart or task list. But even if you're not quite there yet, give yourself a pat on the back for any ground you've gained. (You'll find some rewards for doing well later.) You can continue to work on those tasks in the coming weeks until they are yours for good.

Your efforts as a scientist or investigative reporter should have given you plenty of data on how you're doing during each task: when and where OCD still beats you in that situation, how long it takes for the fear or discomfort to ease, which OCD rule-breaking method is most effective for you, and which tools work best in which circumstances. You already know that the tools in the book have to be adapted to your particular circumstances. How did your creativity help you out in making the program work for you? Were you able to be creative and inventive and have fun thinking up ways to beat OCD at its own game? Are there new OCD hiccups that you need to add to your chart?

What if things didn't go so well? All the problems we've talked about during earlier steps could be at work. Maybe you're bailing out of the task before giving your fear temperature a chance to drop. For OCD to get the message from you, you

Does your fear temperature *have* to go down to 0 or 1 for a situation to be in your territory? Ideally, yes, and that's what you should always be aiming for. But some people are just a little anxious by nature and always will be. If you always seem to be able to get down to a 1 or a 2, and if at that temperature you can go about your business without worrying that OCD is in the way, you can probably consider those symptoms in your territory.

have to let your fear temperature go up when you start a task and hang in there until it drops down to 0 or 1. Maybe you've substituted one ritual for another without realizing it. Really make an effort to tackle OCD with as much enthusiasm and creativity as you can muster. If you can't figure out from your notes what might have gone wrong and what you can do differently, now is a critical time to get help from a therapist. There's no point in launching into this 6-week intermediate phase without the best possible chance of success!

The idea is always to go up the task ladder as fast as you can do it successfully—no slower and no faster. If you're stuck, try dropping down the list a little bit. Maybe you need to modify a task to give it a slightly lower fear temperature. Tackle that first and you may be surprised by how quickly you'll get back to the task that was causing you so much trouble such a short time ago.

Post the summary of Step 6 on your closet door or wherever you'll see it often. This is a long step, so you might need extra cues to keep you on track. Keep your spiral notebook on hand and be sure to transfer any important comments from it to the symptoms on your chart every few days.

Get Going

Set Up Rewards, Notifications, and Ceremonies to Celebrate Successes

Many kids are so thrilled to find themselves breaking free as they take back more and more territory from OCD that they wouldn't think of asking for a reward for their achievements. Freedom from OCD is reward enough. Or, if you and your parents were having a rough time over OCD before you started this program, you might feel that you owe it to your family to get better rather than that anyone owes you a special treat for doing so. The truth is, however, that everyone appreciates rewards to keep at a tough task. This is hard work and takes time and dedication that is worth recognizing. Also, a ceremony, notification, or reward is a way of saying publicly how far you've come. Without marking your milestones, it's easy to lose track of how much progress you've actually made. Just think back to where you were a few weeks ago and you'll see the truth of this statement!

What are rewards, ceremonies, and notifications?

A *reward* is something nice that you get to recognize that you've made progress in your goals. It can be a simple as a compliment or as big as a new car. It is not being paid for doing homework (although that, too, is OK for some kids)—it is the recognition that there is merit in the hard work you put into facing OCD instead of running from it.

A *ceremony* is a reward that takes the form of a party—something from your parents like "Hey, let's go have pizza tonight" or "How would you like to have some friends over for a movie?"

A *notification* is a special kind of ceremony designed to let people you've had problems with or felt awkward around because of OCD know that it was OCD that was the problem and that now you're on top of it instead of its being on top of you. For example, you might want to let a special friend or a grandparent know that you really do like him or her but couldn't show it until now because OCD was in the way.

Though you can always reward yourself—giving yourself a pat on the back is a good thing to practice—perhaps the best way to work out rewards is to do it with your parents, especially if they think you ought to just get rid of OCD on your own. Sit down at dinner or some other time when you're all together—your brothers and sisters can be included, too, because they'll likely be on hand for ceremonies if not for all the rewards—and do a little brainstorming. You'll need to decide on how often a reward or ceremony should be awarded and what it will be. You might want to designate small rewards for individual achievements, such as adding a symptom to your territory, and then assign ceremonies for the big milestones, such as cutting the size of your symptom list by 20%. A reward can be something as simple as getting to pick the video your family is going to rent or something more elaborate, like a family day at an amusement park.

Ceremonies can be planned or spontaneous. Set a goal; plan a ceremony. Or, at the end of a tough week in which you made a lot of progress but are tired from the effort, a simple dinner out with friends or family can be a really nice way of recognizing what you've done. A ceremony can take place at the local McDonald's, where your family all applauds you for your accomplishments, or it can be a more involved party, where friends and extended family all cheer you for what you've achieved.

A notification is similar to a ceremony, but it means just telling others about the territory you've taken back from OCD. Of course, not everyone needs to know about OCD, but if you're like most kids there will be some people that you want to know probably because you've been avoiding them or they've been avoiding you because of OCD. Having problems getting along with people you care about because of OCD can really hurt, and that hurt can rob you of the energy you need to keep up your good work against OCD. Notifications take on this problem.

Sometimes we print up fancy little cards or cardboard plaques for kids to send to selected cheerleaders, such as grandparents and teachers. Or a notification can be as simple as calling Grandma to announce a new victory over OCD or sending an e-mail message to your teacher. What ties rewards, ceremonies, and notifications together is positive feelings: Anything that makes you feel good about your progress is appropriate for one of these celebrations. And anything that your parents think is practical and reasonable among those choices is just fine.

Once you've decided on what you'll do and when, you can make up a list of specific rewards, notifications, and ceremonies to post where you'll see it to keep you going. Put it right next to your summary of the step you're working on so you'll see it all the time.

Start Intermediate Tasks

You have 4 to 6 weeks of "intermediate" tasks ahead of you, and you'll find you can accomplish a lot in this time. Instead of one OCD hiccup at a time, you're going to tackle several. However, your first task is to remap OCD. Take a look at your symptom chart. How has your territory grown and OCD's shrunk? Eliminate any symptoms you've conquered and make sure that any new ones that you and your parents have discovered in the last few weeks are added. Redefine your work zone. Undoubtedly some tasks that caused you significant anxiety (say a 7 or 8) are now only a 4 or 5 or so, and you can consider those as EX/RP targets for the weeks ahead.

> When I got started on the program, it was so easy I thought I could do anything. I touched stuff, stopped praying and checking, and just went wacko stopping stuff in the work zone. I felt great until I started trying harder stuff. I never did get all the way to zero again, but I always got at least to 1 or 2, and that was enough to keep OCD from bothering me.
> —Patty, age 15

With your parents' support, choose two, maybe even three, new tasks for the coming week. Some will take all week, doing EX/RP every day, to finally nail. Others will be gone in a few days. Give yourself 2 days on easy EX/RP, with temperatures that don't go up with exposure, so you can be confident that the stop signal for a particular hiccup is probably fixed. If it comes back, nail it again right away. Talk about how you plan to break OCD's rules if you don't think you can completely stop a particular ritual. Take one hiccup and break it down into a ladder of its own, and then take on every bit of OCD that sits in the work zone, working your way up to the harder stuff over the next week or two. Also discuss which of your tools you plan to rely on for each task.

You've reached an important transition, as we said earlier in the chapter. It's time to acknowledge that you're beginning to really be in charge now. You've done your trial tasks; you know you can beat OCD a little at a time; you know what tools are your best allies; and you know the signs of trouble that should make you slow down, take stock, preserve your gains, and maintain your momentum. In fact, this point in your work probably calls for a ceremony with family or friends!

While you're celebrating with your family, take the opportunity to discuss the role your parents should play from now on. So far they've been mainly cheerleaders. They should have been gently coaxing you forward without telling you what to do, scolding you for perceived "failures," or pushing you too fast. But you've been in charge. That's where we want you to stay, but we also want you to take full advantage of what your parents have learned by this point. By observing your progress and seeing what works and doesn't work for you, your parents have become pretty knowledgeable about OCD, and if you want them to, they can begin to be more active in helping you make progress. Is there a place where you could start to let your parents withdraw from participating in your rituals? Is there anything else your parents could do to help that they haven't been doing so far? For example:

- If you rely on your mom to speed you up so you won't be late when OCD has you doing rituals, ask her not to.
- If your parents help with checking rituals, give them the day off.
- If your mom or dad answers OCD's questions over and over, give yourself and them a budget: You can spend so many questions and that's it.
- If you rely on reassurance, ask them not to reassure you.
- If OCD makes your parents buy stuff (such as cleaning supplies), do extra driving (to a "safe" restaurant), or not go places (say, out to dinner), try to break these rules—it'll make your parents happy, and that's a good thing.

Try strategizing how you might do this, but remember that it has to be completely open, honest, based on kindness, and low in the work zone, so that you don't end up fighting.

Terrible Trouble says my mommy has to say goodbye five times or she will be in an accident and maybe die and it will be my fault. Sometimes she has to say it five times five times in a row. She gets kind of mad, but I get real scared and call her from school, which is worse. But I did it. I told her to only say goodbye four times, and I didn't call even though I got scared. By the end of the week we were down to two. Yes!

—Rodrigo, age 8

OCD was a real terror in my family, especially for my mom, who had to wash the dishes in a certain way, sometimes more than once. Well, we agreed that this had to stop, which we did one dish at a time. The bad news is now I have to do the dishes, but that's OK because my grandma doesn't think I'm lazy anymore. That ceremony of notification was really cool.

—Amy, age 16

This is also a good time to see whether you want to get anyone else involved. If you have a mature sibling, a supportive grandparent, a good friend, or even a teacher who you think could function in the same way your parents have, or at least as an "advanced" cheerleader, talk about assigning that person a bigger role. Could this relative help you simply with a new level of cheerleading and support? How about with reminders to use your toolkit and to keep breaking OCD's rules? Be careful here; you don't want to ask people to be involved to the point of making you feel as if you're constantly being monitored by everyone you know. But this is a good time to figure out how you can take advantage of all your resources, especially if some of them are also involved in OCD.

I couldn't go over to my friend Susie's because she had a pet bird and OCD had me really worried about the bird flu and getting me and my mom sick. We talked about it, and I set up a "bird chart" that started with going into the backyard and ended up holding the damn bird. That was hard, but it worked. No more bird flu fears, and Susie and I can hang out at her house again.

—Melanie, age 15

I quit spending the night at my uncle Bill's because Dumbbutt made me do certain things every morning in my room. I don't know why except that I felt like I wouldn't have a good day unless I cleaned and straightened up in a certain way. Not seeing my uncle was a drag; we like to go fishing. My dad was always too busy with work to fish. Uncle Bill thought I was mad at him until we talked about DumbButt. He came over and helped me clobber DumbButt one morning. After that, we went fishing. Now I can go to his house again. Once my dad came as a reward for me. I hope he comes again. We had fun.

—Allan, age 9

Among other things, OCD made me worry that if I looked at another girl I was a lesbian. I like guys. Pretty soon I couldn't be around my girlfriends, and then I couldn't even look at my mom. Everyone thought I was weird. I thought I was weird—heck, OCD is weird. It felt so good to tell my best friend about this. With Mom, we figured out how to start at the mall looking at girls I didn't know, and then I graduated to friends. Mom came last. The best part was my dad and my stupid brother never knew about this one. I'd have been so embarrassed.

—Sue, age 15

I used to worry—sorry, OCD made me worry—that if I had a bad thought, I would go to hell and maybe my parents, too. My dad helped me talk to my priest about this—he said that OCD is an illness and not to worry about God, who just wants me to get well. He even helped me work out how to stop some of the prayers and said he wanted to be sure I stayed with my confirmation classes.

—Ben, age 10

At this point you can extend the work zone to one item that is a 4 or even a 5 on the symptom chart or task list, but only if you're successful enough at resisting to think you can be 100% successful. Be modest in your goals, but don't underestimate what you can do. Pay attention to how you do and pick up the pace if you're doing really well. You might find that you're able to eliminate one or more of the tasks you've picked before the end of the week. Or you might notice that, without planning to do so, you're working on other symptoms, too. If either of those things happens, next week you can try stepping things up in one of two ways: (1) add another task or two so that you're working on more tasks during the week or (2) move a little (not a lot) more quickly up the fear thermometer.

What you'll probably find is that you're doing a lot of resisting of OCD symptoms that you haven't listed as specific targets. This is a very good sign. It means that you're getting the idea that this program works, and so OCD is losing its power over you. Be careful to stay within the work zone, however. It's easy here to take a giant step backward if you get too ambitious and find yourself bailing out on a task because you bit off more than you could chew. Also, before you quit doing a specific EX/RP homework task, make sure that you've really nailed it; no getting ahead of yourself, as that's just playing into OCD's hands.

At the beginning of each new week, assess your progress. Do this at another family meeting if you all agree that family meetings are part of the program or just with one parent or on your own, depending on what's best for you. Take a look at your symptom chart and your task lists. What can you eliminate? Is there anything you need to add?

For teenagers: You can definitely try going it alone if you're comfortable doing so at this point. But be sure to agree to a weekly meeting with your parents so they can see what kind of progress you're making—and so they can celebrate it along with you! Try not to let your pride get in the way of your victory over OCD. If you see that you're not making as steady progress as you were with fuller participation from your parents, ask them to step in and help again for another week. You can always try to go it alone again after that. Don't judge your progress—just do the best you can doing your homework every day. We live in an achievement-oriented society in which there's tremendous pressure to excel. Be realistic about OCD—you are doing the best you can in any given moment.

Consider Letting Your Parents Select a Situation for a Task

This goal can take two different forms. If, as you discussed during Step 5, your parents are entangled in your rituals—as some but not all parents are—together you can agree on one ritual for Mom and Dad to stop cooperating with. (Rodrigo and Amy, and maybe you, too, started doing this in baby steps, as described earlier, before 4 weeks of Step 6 were up.) Or, if your parents aren't involved in your rituals, you can consider letting them pick next week's targets for you from the work zone based on what's important to them (if they haven't already been helping you pick your target symptoms).

To do either, you need to feel comfortable that your parents now understand OCD and their role in helping you beat it. If OCD caused any conflict between you and your parents, it should be mostly gone. In addition, you should be able to view your parents as your main cheerleaders—loving adults you can count on to remind you of all of your victories over OCD so far and of all the good things about you that have nothing to do with your battle with OCD. If you've reached that point, your parents can take a more active role in helping you win the fight, because now you can be sure they'll be totally positive and helpful and you won't worry about whether they're going to push you too fast because they hate seeing you upset by OCD.

Guidelines for Working Your Way Through Intermediate Tasks

As you sit down to work out the sequence of tasks to target from the work zone, remember these things and keep them in mind as you do the tasks themselves:

1. You've come a very long way in a short time. Change is possible—you've proven it already.
2. Change happened because you changed your view of yourself in relationship to OCD and then changed how you relate to OCD by doing the opposite of what it asks of you. Remember that it's just a meaningless hiccup. When you get anxious or upset, anchor yourself in your body by focusing on your breathing or some other physical sensation that seems appropriate, look around to remind yourself what's actually happening, and tell yourself that "OCD is just a nonsense hiccup—it'll pass just like the weather. All I need to do is something other than what OCD asks of me and it'll go away."
3. Use whatever language works best to put OCD in its proper place. In doing so, practice being kind to yourself. No need to beat yourself up about OCD. You didn't ask for it—and you are doing the best you can to face it directly.
4. Remind yourself that OCD is not the enemy; it is believing in OCD and going along with it that is the enemy. Don't take responsibility for what makes no sense.
5. If you find yourself asking "Is this OCD?" or "Am I a bad person?" and then getting stuck trying to figure out the answer, this is OCD, not you.
6. Once you've committed to a task, see it through. Bailing out is the best way there is to give power back to OCD. It says "I believe in what you say" and "I can't do anything but what you tell me." Although at least the second part may still be true in part for stuff that's way up there on your chart, you'll get there step by step until OCD isn't hiccupping anymore. But you have to see it through—no one can do this but you.

We generally think it's best not to tackle this goal until you've done 4 weeks of Step 6, but some kids try it earlier if they're doing really well at their chosen tasks for the step. Or they break down a ritual that involves Mom or Dad into tiny little bits and have Mom or Dad start backing out of the ritual. Like everything else, this is a place where creativity can really help drive the program forward, so have fun with your folks figuring out how to take on OCD together.

If your parents are not entangled in OCD, tell them that you'd like them to pick a target for you for the coming week. (Limit it to one even if you're going to work on more than one this week, so that you can try this out gradually.) The idea is that your parents will find some rituals more troublesome for the family than others, and now you're giving them the chance to pick one that they would like to eliminate from everyone's life—as long as it has a fear temperature that puts it in the work zone. Understand that the symptom they pick may not be the one you would choose. That's what makes this part of Step 6 different: You're turning a little more of the control over OCD to your parents than you have so far. You can do this now because you've clearly established that you're the expert and you're in charge of beating OCD. Letting your parents get a little more involved won't rob you of that control.

When I say that you're turning over a little more control to your parents, however, I mean only that you're giving them a chance to participate in target selection in a way that they haven't before. You still have to agree to their choice. If you feel that you can't work on this symptom this week, say so in no uncertain terms. Ask if they can pick another one or, if not, try inviting them to make a choice again next week, when you might feel differently.

If your parents are tangled up in OCD rituals, see if you can all agree on one in which your parents can stop cooperating with OCD. Let's say OCD tells you that if you're not absolutely certain that all the doors are locked, a burglar will break into your house and hurt someone in your family. OCD tells you that you have to go through elaborate lock-checking routines to make sure this doesn't happen. Your parents have been trying to help ease your mind by doing a lot of the checking for you, but you know it's really hard on them to do it day after day. When you invite them to stop participating in one of the lock-checking rituals, they choose the bedtime ritual, in which one of them goes through the house in a particular order, unlocking and relocking every door, repeats the route three more times, then tells you everything is locked tight and you can turn your light out. The idea of trying to sleep without the reassurance of your nighttime ritual terrifies you, so you say you don't think you're ready to tackle that target yet. But you don't leave it there. You suggest you might be able to handle it if, instead, your parents stop the daytime routine of getting out of the car in the driveway and pulling on the garage door to make sure that the remote control did in fact shut the door tightly before driving away. Your mom says that would be great, adding with a laugh, "I hate it when Mr. N [your name for OCD, the N standing for Nervous] makes me dodge raindrops in my own driveway anyway." You all agree you'll try this for a week and, if you're able to beat Mr. N in the driveway, you'll work your way up slowly to the nighttime unlocking and locking ritual, perhaps dropping one door at a time.

Now you and your parents need to discuss how you plan to talk back to OCD to get through the fear you will feel at first when you leave home without having Mom or Dad check the garage door. Which of your tools might work best? If the fear thermometer goes up really high and stays there for longer than you can take, what OCD rule-breaking method could you use to wean yourself from relying on your parents to check the door? All of you must be as candid as possible about the reactions you might have to trying this new routine. In what ways is it likely that you might try to avoid the whole thing? Brainstorm potential reactions and plan how you'll react. Have fun. Maybe you can all agree, for example, that if you say "I think I'll ride my bike today" when Mom heads for the garage and says it's time to leave for soccer practice, Mom will make a joke about the fact that she'd rather beat Mr. N than save a fraction of a gallon of gas. Or maybe you can agree on a code phrase for Mom or Dad to use to ask in a kind way whether you're really sick or just trying to avoid having to get in the car to go out—such as "Your idea or Mr. N's?"

Taking Stock

Feeling a little stronger? How about *a lot* stronger? Many kids like to draw a new picture of their "land" at this point to show how much bigger their territory is getting than it was before—and how much smaller OCD's has become. Use the OCD scale and graph your progress; then, if you want, go ahead and draw a map like the one on page 121 that you think shows what your territory looks like now that you've finished Step 6. Look at your "Getting Stronger Every Day" form and give yourself a loud "Way to go!" for doing all that work over the past 6 weeks. And now . . . anyone for a pizza party?

At the end of each day, check off whether you've followed the instructions for Step 6 (and Step 7 once you move forward to it), spending 30–60 minutes a day. This chart allows 5 weeks for Steps 6 and 7, but if you need more time on these steps, add the extra days using your own paper.

Day 36 ☐ I did the homework for Step 6. ☐ I did the homework for Step 7.

Day 37 ☐ I did the homework for Step 6. ☐ I did the homework for Step 7.

Day 38 ☐ I did the homework for Step 6. ☐ I did the homework for Step 7.

Day 39 ☐ I did the homework for Step 6. ☐ I did the homework for Step 7.

Day 40 ☐ I did the homework for Step 6. ☐ I did the homework for Step 7.

Day 41 ☐ I did the homework for Step 6. ☐ I did the homework for Step 7.

Day 42 ☐ I did the homework for Step 6. ☐ I did the homework for Step 7.

Day 43 ☐ I did the homework for Step 6. ☐ I did the homework for Step 7.

Day 44 ☐ I did the homework for Step 6. ☐ I did the homework for Step 7.

Day 45 ☐ I did the homework for Step 6. ☐ I did the homework for Step 7.

Day 46 ☐ I did the homework for Step 6. ☐ I did the homework for Step 7.

Day 47 ☐ I did the homework for Step 6. ☐ I did the homework for Step 7.

Day 48 ☐ I did the homework for Step 6. ☐ I did the homework for Step 7.

Day 49 ☐ I did the homework for Step 6. ☐ I did the homework for Step 7.

Day 50 ☐ I did the homework for Step 6. ☐ I did the homework for Step 7.

Day 51 ☐ I did the homework for Step 6. ☐ I did the homework for Step 7.

Day 52 ☐ I did the homework for Step 6. ☐ I did the homework for Step 7.

Day 53 ☐ I did the homework for Step 6. ☐ I did the homework for Step 7.

(cont.)

Day 54 ☐ I did the homework for Step 6. ☐ I did the homework for Step 7.

Day 55 ☐ I did the homework for Step 6. ☐ I did the homework for Step 7.

Day 56 ☐ I did the homework for Step 6. ☐ I did the homework for Step 7.

Day 57 ☐ I did the homework for Step 6. ☐ I did the homework for Step 7.

Day 58 ☐ I did the homework for Step 6. ☐ I did the homework for Step 7.

Day 59 ☐ I did the homework for Step 6. ☐ I did the homework for Step 7.

Day 60 ☐ I did the homework for Step 6. ☐ I did the homework for Step 7.

Day 61 ☐ I did the homework for Step 6. ☐ I did the homework for Step 7.

Day 62 ☐ I did the homework for Step 6. ☐ I did the homework for Step 7.

Day 63 ☐ I did the homework for Step 6. ☐ I did the homework for Step 7.

Day 64 ☐ I did the homework for Step 6. ☐ I did the homework for Step 7.

Day 65 ☐ I did the homework for Step 6. ☐ I did the homework for Step 7.

Day 66 ☐ I did the homework for Step 6. ☐ I did the homework for Step 7.

Day 67 ☐ I did the homework for Step 6. ☐ I did the homework for Step 7.

Day 68 ☐ I did the homework for Step 6. ☐ I did the homework for Step 7.

Day 69 ☐ I did the homework for Step 6. ☐ I did the homework for Step 7.

Day 70 ☐ I did the homework for Step 6. ☐ I did the homework for Step 7.

Step 6: Instructions for Parents

IN ESSENCE this step and the next one form the core of the program. Your child knows the ropes and will now devote the next 1 to 3 months to eliminating all the OCD symptoms on his chart. Because this step takes 4 to 6 weeks, it's easy to get off track or let the program take second place to other priorities. Life happens, and it is always tempting to rush off to the store or soccer or the dentist or whatever and skip the EX/RP homework. Doing EX/RP at the high end of the work zone is hard work—no question about it. You have to be committed to make the program work. No matter how old or sick the child with OCD, you can be a big help in preventing "days off" from EX/RP. As we've said before, steady progress is key to maintaining gains. To help your child stay motivated, your job will be to offer a combination of reminders about what's on the agenda and celebrations of what he's achieved. This can be a tricky balance. Be sure your nudges are gentle but consistent and that the rewards, too, are delivered on a regular basis and *always* for real accomplishments, never because you think your child just needs a boost in mood or confidence. (This is not to say that you shouldn't give your child a boost when he's feeling low or unsure of himself in general; just don't tie it to OCD. There are so many other great areas of your child's life, so many great aspects of him, to focus on.)

To keep your child going with the program, try making statements and asking questions like these:

- "Wow, I just noticed from your 'Getting Stronger . . .' form that you've already done a whole week of Step 6. Way to go! What do you think has gone well? Need any help?"
- At bedtime: "You seemed to have a pretty [tough, successful, hard, frustrating—whatever you've observed] day with OCD. Don't forget to check off all that work you did today!"

- "Hey, tomorrow's Saturday. Don't forget our family meeting at breakfast. If it's time for a reward, we can figure out then what it should be."
- "I noticed you were pretty quiet about Germy yesterday, but I didn't see you doing a lot of washing. Did you write down any thoughts in your notebook?"

How much structure you want to apply to this step will have a lot to do with your child's age and inclinations. Limit yourself to coaching with statements like those above if your child is determined to go it alone and capable of doing so. In that case you'll want to observe very closely to make sure the child isn't losing ground. For kids who benefit from more structure in most things they do, from chores to homework to play, feel free to come up with your own calendars that note when family meetings will be held, when you'll review the week's work and draw up a new work zone on the symptom chart, and any other regular events that will help keep your child on track. Use stickers or other symbols to make the calendar visually appealing. Or try using a white board where you post funny little cheers and reminders for your child. Combine weekly reviews with notifications to make all these events fun. You could, for example, schedule a regular call to Grandma after your weekly review of the symptom chart, telling her all about what your child has achieved, and then follow it with a small celebration such as making waffles for Sunday brunch.

Get Ready

Reviewing Step 5 is the most important preparation for Step 6. Some parents have a hard time determining what success at Step 5 really looks like. This is especially true if your child has had a hard time getting the fear temperature all the way down to 0 during tasks. You'll have to think about the bigger picture here (and watch what happens on the tasks in Step 6). Maybe your child is still a little anxious at the end of each task. But can she fully participate in whatever she's doing despite this anxiety? Does she stay with response prevention without bailing out? Would you say that, even if she's still a little anxious, she has been able to return to her daily activities without being preoccupied or derailed even a little bit by OCD? If so, think about your child's temperament. Would you describe her as nervous or high-strung in general? If that's just part of her personality, the key in assessing success with EX/RP tasks will always be whether OCD is still getting in her way. If it's not, getting the fear temperature down to 1, and maybe even 2 on the situations that caused the most discomfort to begin with, could be enough.

   If, on the other hand, you believe your child is having a hard time truly eliminating the tasks she's tried so far, help her review what went wrong. Look through her notebook together. Or ask her if you can record the fear temperatures she reports during a few practice tasks so you can tell whether her anxiety is actually rising as it's supposed to and then falling as it should. If not, you'll have to figure out why not. Usually, the reason is that the task turned out to be too hard, so all you need to do is to break it down into something more manageable. For example, if your child has trouble stopping a washing ritual, cut back on time or find some other way to break the rule on day 1, something else on day 2, until on day 7 he can stop washing altogether.

If everything you've read so far doesn't help you turn up an answer, talk to a therapist. You and your child's therapist should also keep close track of how much time it takes your child to get through Steps 6 and 7. You can allow up to 5 months for the whole program, but any more than that will be counterproductive. So you can add up to 8 more weeks for Steps 6 and 7 than is shown on the "Getting Stronger Every Day" form if necessary. But if progress is stalled, extra time won't necessarily be the answer.

Here are a few other possibilities to consider if your child doesn't seem to be conquering symptoms at a steady pace:

• *Does your child need an incentive to do the homework to begin with?* Some particularly active, busy kids have a hard time fitting in the 30–60 minutes of "homework" that they're supposed to do every day. If this seems to be the case for your child, you may actually have to set up a reward system not just for elimination of symptoms from the symptom chart but also for checking off the completion of EX/RP homework every day. If you do this, make sure it's very clear to your child exactly what you consider the minimum effort he needs to invest to earn the reward: just 30 minutes, 45 minutes, or the full 60? Exactly what do you expect him to do? Many parents find it helpful to draw up an informal but written contract to spell all this out so that everyone has something to refer back to. And, in Step 6, when you review each week's accomplishments, you should also review this contract to see whether it needs revision for the coming week.

• *Have you been able to distinguish between undesirable behavior connected with OCD and that connected to just being a kid?* Let's say your child has an obsession about burglars that makes everyone have to check locks repeatedly before he feels comfortable turning off the light and going to bed. One of the tasks he's been practicing involves cutting down on the time spent on these bedtime rituals. He's had mixed success over the past week. Are you sure his efforts to postpone bedtime are always connected with OCD-stimulated fears? Maybe he's done better against OCD than you think—but he just felt like staying up a little later on a couple of nights. We're not suggesting your child is manipulating you (though kids certainly do that sometimes). Rather, you may have simply jumped to conclusions when your child begged for a few more minutes before the light was turned out.

To make sure they understand what is OCD and what is the child, some parents and their children simply agree that when parents have any doubts, they will ask, and the children will answer honestly. You might use your child's nickname for OCD and ask whether, for example, Sneaky is making your child afraid to turn out the light. If he says yes, you reply with sympathy. If not, you react the way you would when any of your kids tries to stall over bedtime. If this tactic doesn't seem to work for you, especially if oppositional behavior has been a persistent problem independent of OCD, you probably need to consult a therapist.

• *Is your child motivated to eliminate his compulsions?* What if your son hates his first-period class at school, and lining up his books over and over in his room before he leaves for school often gets him out of that class? Or what if your daughter, who has contamination obsessions, gets out of doing all housecleaning chores as a result? If your child doesn't seem to be making the effort you'd expect to conquer certain symptoms, you'll have to give serious thought to whether she gets something from performing the rituals. In that case, you have a couple of choices. First, with your child's consent, you can establish a consequence for not working at the task that will outweigh any benefit gained. If your son doesn't want to stop missing his first period, you could have him miss out on a certain amount of after-school play time on days when he does miss the first period because of obeying OCD. If your daughter hates math, you and she can assign extra math problems if EX/RP homework isn't done. This is not punishment, but a consensual way of increasing motivation to confront OCD. Be careful here. You absolutely don't want to get into a pattern of punishments surrounding this program. The second choice is to make sure your child doesn't escape normal responsibilities by adding a task that she can handle that is equivalent to the one nixed by OCD. If she can't handle cleaning chores right now, give her the responsibility for household chores that will take just as much time. If she knows she won't get out of chores, there won't be anything to be gained in holding on to contamination fears.

Get Going

Set Up Rewards, Notifications, and Ceremonies to Celebrate Successes

It's important that your system for rewards, notifications, and ceremonies be devised by all of you together. If these are your ideas and aren't too appealing to your child, they won't be a very strong positive reinforcement. On the other hand, some parents get carried away. They are so relieved to see their child making progress and so eager to be able to respond to the child positively that they overdo it. Giving a child a new computer for deleting one symptom from his list, for example, leaves you nowhere to go for later, bigger accomplishments. (This is also the reason that it's wise to set up a whole hierarchy of rewards now, rather than assigning a reward for a recent accomplishment and planning to decide on the next reward when the time comes.) Rewards do not equal bribes. It is a tough job tackling OCD—that's why we call it the work zone—and for some kids, paying them for doing extra "chores" is just the ticket to motivate and reward them for doing what needs to be done to complete the program. Just remember that the rewards, ceremonies, and notifications are strictly for positive reinforcement of something the child has already achieved. They are not to be used as bribes or to coerce the child into doing something that he or she is not yet ready for. Be cautious also about the extent to which your child might see rewards as pressures to perform—remember that the best reward is always no more OCD. Make sure that the reward follows successful EX/RP—that way it is truly a reward and maintains the essential motivational ingredient in the program: "I need to do EX/RP to get my brain to stop hiccupping."

Helping younger kids: Younger kids may need a little more guidance in coming up with rewards. Better to give very young kids a selection of ideas to choose from than to make the choices open-ended, which might lead to overly grand selections and, when you have to reject them, disappointment—another form of punishment. Also be aware that younger kids benefit from more frequent reinforcement, so come up with little rewards and ceremonies for more modest, but predictably more regular, accomplishments.

Helping teenagers: The scope of reward here must be more under the control of your teen. Teens often propose something surprising, or perhaps not: money, clothes, CDs, and time with friends are always popular. Just make sure that the scope of the reward matches both your teen's need for reinforcement (some teens require more in the way of high-salience rewards than others) and your sense of what is proportionate to the effort expended.

How a therapist can help: Brainstorming and cooperative decision making come more easily to some families than to others. If you just can't seem to come to agreement on rewards, notifications, and ceremonies, enlist the aid of a therapist to serve as coach (or referee!). This is particularly true when there is conflict in the extended family over whether OCD is a real illness and about how it should be managed. If you and your spouse are at odds regarding OCD, and this conflict spreads into the extended family, a therapist skilled at helping everyone get on the same page can be a lifesaver.

Start Intermediate Tasks

If your child does find himself resisting OCD in ways that weren't identified as specific targets—and you may want to ask your child directly every couple of days whether he thinks this is happening—be alert for overly ambitious efforts or tasks that are clearly outside the work zone. It's so easy to take a step back during this stage if your child starts to move too fast. Just because your child can resist in some areas doesn't mean he can just stop doing rituals. In fact, you may need to remind him to slow down and get it right. Practicing patience is a good thing for the first week or two of Step 6. Then it's off to the races for a while for most kids, until they hit the most difficult situations at the top of the symptom chart, when things tend to slow down again.

If your child is agreeing to a new level of participation from you, be deferential. This is not the time to step in and exercise excessive control over your child's progress. In fact, some older children and teenagers will wish to take over full responsibility for their own EX/RP tasks at this point. Becoming independent is a critical part of their development, and even if you feel some trepidation about letting them loose this way, let them try it if they want to. Recapping how the week went at your weekly family meeting will reveal whether this new tactic is working and, if not, how it can be modified to allow your child to continue to pursue autonomy without giving up progress toward beating OCD. In our family, there was a time when my teens saw a family meeting as a punishment, and I suppose to them it was. Don't push it unless it makes sense.

Helping younger kids: The key at this point is consistency. The younger they are, the more likely it may be that kids will lose interest in their EX/RP program and want to stop working so hard. Besides sticking with them as they do their EX/RP homework, you'll need to call into play all the positive reinforcement you can come up with to keep them going. If this means increasing the incentives by redoing your rewards hierarchy or adding more frequent ceremonies and notifications, don't hesitate to do so. Just don't let their lack of interest lead to laxity in the form of taking the easy route and picking EX/RP targets that are too easy. You'll have a hint that this is happening if progress up the symptom chart slows.

How a therapist can help: If you're not sure where you stand at this point, for whatever reason (the child's progress varies widely from week to week, your teenager has become tight-lipped and you really can't tell what's going on, etc.), you're likely stuck and will need the help of a therapist to get unstuck. Put differently, if everyone isn't with the program and happy to be doing better, you'll probably need experienced help to make the kind of progress you all hope for.

Select a Situation for a Task

This goal is a big temptation for a lot of parents. If OCD makes your child do rituals that have been causing you lots of trouble and inconvenience, you undoubtedly want to make them history as soon as possible. Don't let your enthusiasm lead you on here. First, we suggest not tackling this goal until the first month of Step 6 has passed. If your child is doing so well that she seems very confident before then, you can very gently ask whether she feels ready to add this goal to her homework. But if he or she hesitates, back off immediately and tell her you'll revisit the idea after week 4.

When you do get to this goal, remember that your child must agree to the goal you choose. To avoid the impression that you're putting pressure on her to do something she may not be ready to do, purposely do *not* pick the symptom that you find the biggest hassle for you but one that you can live with for a while longer. In fact, you might consider preparing for this goal by reviewing your child's symptom chart on your own every week and privately identifying three symptoms that you'd like to see her tackle. Then suggest the one that you're least invested in eliminating first.

If your child wants you to help with a ritual "just one more time" after you've picked a task for him to work on, sometimes all you'll need to do is to encourage your child to use his toolkit and remind him of what you all agreed to about this ritual. Also, make sure you and your child's other parent are in agreement about becoming disentangled from OCD. If you end up playing "good cop, bad cop," with one of you giving in to pleas to "help" and the other one resisting, your child will end up feeling it's his fault when a task fails, and that will be a setback.

How a therapist can help: Because this is a new step in parent–child cooperation, it might help to speak to your therapist during the middle of the first week in which you try this, just to report how everything is going. In fact, a weekly phone call to your therapist, if you have one, might be a good idea throughout Step 6, especially if you're having trouble getting organized.

Taking Stock

The whole goal during this step is to keep at it. Progress should be rapid, with all of you feeling that you've turned an important corner. If your child and the rest of the family don't feel this way, then getting professional help is a good idea.

6

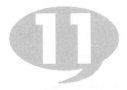

Step 7: Eliminating OCD Everywhere

GO TO THE HEAD OF THE CLASS—you just finished 6 weeks of important work! Let's keep up the momentum.

The Game Plan for Step 7

After reviewing Step 6, do the reading and other preparation listed under "Get Ready" and then plan on spending 6 weeks (or as much time as necessary) following the instructions for this step. This is the second of your two big runs on territory controlled by OCD. You've gone pretty high up the task list and symptom chart and probably have only a few more EX/RP tasks to tackle. Six weeks from now, if all went well, your OCD map should look entirely different than it did before you started this program. Essentially, it will consist of one big circle representing your territory, with OCD nowhere in sight. As always, check off the completion of your homework on your "Getting Stronger Every Day" chart (included at the end of Step 6, Chapter 10). Doing this is particularly helpful to keep you on track during these longer steps in the program.

Get Ready

You did an incredible amount of hard work during Step 6. Congratulations! Your symptom list is proof of how much you've accomplished. It's undoubtedly much shorter than it used to be, and the situations, actions, and triggers that you once rated at 10+ on your fear thermometer now probably get only a 6-8, maybe even less.

This doesn't mean that everything is now a piece of cake, however. In fact, you may have started to feel that your progress began to slow as you worked up the symptom list. Maybe you made short work of two or three different hiccups during the first week or two of Step 6, but by the last week you felt lucky just to eliminate one. That's to be expected and shouldn't discourage you. You're approaching what OCD tells you is the hardest stuff, and the first goal of Step 7 is to help you strengthen what you've gained and then move on to the final goal of getting rid of OCD altogether.

By the way, what OCD says isn't true—the reality is that there isn't any ladder that you have to work your way up. The idea that the top is harder than the bottom is just another bit of OCD, but it probably doesn't feel that way, which is why we try to stay in the work zone as much as possible. If you want to see the truth of this, try dropping the idea that not just OCD but any unwanted thought is somehow part of you. By part of you, I mean that which has anything to do with your personal truth. Identify with the you that is watching, not engaging in story telling. When OCD shows up, relax and pay attention to what is actually happening, accept that OCD is present, *do not* identify OCD as personal in any way even to the point of dropping any story you might hold about OCD, and just go on about your business. After a while, OCD will just fade away. Try the same tactic with other irritations or frustrating desires: Relax and pay attention to what is actually happening, acknowledge what is present, identify with the you that is watching, drop the personal part of the story, and just go on doing the best you can in that moment. Anna really liked gently smiling at OCD and then going on about her business, noting that OCD wasn't really real. She tried the same thing one day when she found herself really mad about something one of her friends had said. She just looked around, took a deep breath, accepted that being mad was present but that nothing bad was happening now and, having let the story go, went on feeling much happier. You might surprise yourself with how much more ease and well-being enters your life when you are not arguing with reality. If this doesn't make sense to you, don't worry about it; just stay with the program as you've been working it.

How did you do with the task your parents chose, or with your choice to allow them to stop cooperating with a ritual? If it went well, you'll give them more freedom to do the same over the next 6 weeks. If you found it really tough, don't worry. One of your other goals for Step 7 is to find ways to let them back away from helping with rituals and instead step forward to help you use your toolkit all the time, everywhere.

If you couldn't eliminate more than one or two hiccups from your list over the past 4 to 6 weeks, now is the time to talk to a therapist about what's holding back your progress. But chances are, if you followed the advice in Chapter 10 and made full use of your parents' support and a therapist's help as needed, you haven't gotten stalled.

Still, some kids think something must be wrong because they've felt their progress slow down. Again, don't get discouraged, and don't be intimidated. You've graduated from the intermediate level and are ready for the "advanced" stage of the program.

Post the summary of Step 7 on your closet door or wherever you'll see it often. This is another long step, so you might need extra cues to keep you on track.

You'll also need lots of help, and you're at the point where you should feel confident that you can count on the support of parents, maybe other relatives, and even a couple of friends. Some kids at this stage have told a close friend or two that they have OCD and have been happy to discover that these true-blue buddies are a huge help in reminding them to use their toolkit. Sometimes the best cheerleaders are your best friends. Just as they'll keep your secrets, defend you, and boost your ego, they'll help you remember that OCD is no match for you.

Keep your notebook on hand and be sure to transfer any important comments from it to the symptoms on your chart every few days.

Get Going

Move Onward and Upward

You know what a plateau is, right? You've been climbing up a steep mountain, getting higher and higher, and suddenly you hit flat ground. It looks like you can't go any higher; your choices are to head back down or stay at the altitude you've already reached. At some point in this program—in fact, often at several points—many kids reach a plateau. You know that one is straight ahead when you feel your progress slowing to a crawl. This feeling may or may not be accompanied by a drop in your enthusiasm to battle OCD or by doubts that you know what to do next.

The most important thing to do when you feel this happening is to tell someone—your parents, your best friend if he or she has been an important source of support, and certainly your therapist if you're working with one. Any of these people, all of whom care very much that you continue to conquer OCD and get back your life, will tell you that this is, if anything, a good sign. It means that you've accomplished a lot and that you're on the verge of a big leap forward.

It may mean that you need a breather—time to rest and consolidate the gains you've made. So take a week off with no new tasks. Don't stop resisting OCD, but very deliberately stop pushing yourself to try something harder, think about how far you've come, and, above all, celebrate. You need to recognize not only that you've accomplished so much but also that you're about to ask more of yourself than ever before. What's ahead of you are the hardest tasks, the ones that fall into a somewhat different realm from what you've tackled so far. These are the tasks that used to be a 10+. They may be only a 5 or 6 by now, though some almost certainly are still a 7 or 8 on your fear thermometer, thanks to all your efforts over the preceding weeks. You and anyone who's on your cheerleading squad needs to recognize in some concrete way that you're about to set out for a whole new level of resisting OCD, one that just a few weeks ago seemed unimaginable. It will be easier than you think, but you still need to go through it. Let's get after it.

So the beginning of Step 7 calls for both a significant celebration and a major pat on the back. (It wouldn't hurt to throw in a special reward, too.) Start by complimenting yourself. You may think you know how far you've come, but let's make sure it really sinks in. Pull out your hiccup chart and any task ladders you've been using. Look carefully at how many items you were able to cross off over the last month. I bet what you erased included some tasks you thought you'd never be able to accomplish, and yet they've vanished from your radar screen. Also notice how few are left. By this time in the program many kids have only three or four items left to eliminate. Just to make sure you really see your progress, redraw your map of OCD (from page 121). Even better, ask your parents to redraw it as they see it. How do you think you'll feel when you see that OCD's territory now looks like an eraser-sized circle while yours looks like a Frisbee? You should feel proud. Of course, then you'll have to figure out what to do with all that free time!

Now go ahead and implement the plan you made at the beginning of Step 6 to celebrate this accomplishment. Here's one time when you might want to revise whatever reward, celebration, and/or notification you planned a month ago. Sometimes reaching this stage proves to be much more meaningful than you or your family could have anticipated. Why? Because by now life should be somewhat easier, if not a lot easier, because there's less OCD around and also because you all know that you can do it. If the celebration you planned now seems kind of flat, pump it up. Be sure that whatever rewards, ceremony, or notification you had in mind really reflect the significance of this turning point.

With my mom's help I got a little bit more than halfway up the symptom chart. I'm ready to do more on my own, which makes her happy. She bought me a new dress, and I wore it to Grandma's when I told her about OCD.

—Angela, age 12

Whoopee, I got my driver's license!

—Robert, age 17

When I got about two-thirds up the symptom chart, I sort of stalled out. The items toward the top all involved someone in my family dying because I forgot to check something. I was pretty discouraged, but my dad reminded me that the program said it would get harder and slow down toward the top. We agreed to go one by one and just knock them off. Each one I get, I get a CD or a videogame.

—Billy Joe, age 16

Hi, Mom. Stinky doesn't like you, so he won't play with me anymore. I don't miss him. He stinks. Can we get messy again and then go for ice cream?

—Mark, age 6

When I got to the upper third of my symptom chart, I got all wrapped up in the idea that these OCD symptoms were harder, and so I got scared and took a week off. That was OK—I needed a rest. But really, the idea of harder is just a story I told myself about OCD. It plays right into OCD's hands. So I tried just watching what is happening without turning it into a story. It was amazing—stuff that I thought was a 10 wasn't much harder than stuff that I rated a 3 or 4. I'm going to be done with this *#%H# before long, and will I be glad!

—Eleanor, age 17

Once you've celebrated, it's time to get back to business. First, take a quick review of what might sink your ship as you move forward.

- Is it possible that you've been adding mental rituals to help you deal with not doing the ritual you've assigned yourself the task of resisting?
- Are you telling yourself that something bad will happen (your dog will get hurt, the house will catch fire, your dad will get sick) if you perform the ritual? If so, add this new ritual to your symptom chart. Better yet, just drop whatever it is you're telling yourself.
- Are you helping yourself get through the discomfort of the task by telling yourself you'll just do it later? That's what OCD wants to hear. Try to be honest with yourself—and your parents or therapist if you need help with this—and add this to your symptom chart.
- If your parents used to get involved in OCD by reassuring you that your obsession wouldn't come true and now you've asked them to stop doing this, are you remembering the way they used to reassure you in your head during the task? It's a natural thing to do, but it means you're substituting for parents and playing by OCD's rules. Add this to your list, too.

If adding these new symptoms to your chart feels discouraging, remember that this is you forcing OCD to crawl out from under its rock, bringing it out in the open where you can deal with it directly. You are now stronger than OCD, whether you believe that 100% of the time or not, and once it's out there in the sunlight, the advantage is yours. Besides, these are generally tasks you'll master more easily than the ones originally on your chart.

You and your parents should sit down and take a good look at your new work zone. How is it different from before? For some kids, the items at the top of the symptom list differ from the ones they've conquered in some significant way. Maybe you can face a bathroom doorknob or some other object that makes you worry about germs at home, at other people's houses, and at school. But you still haven't been able to use a restaurant's restroom or touch a bathroom door in any public place. Or maybe you can deal with your fears about unlocked doors and windows all day and even in the middle of the night when you wake up to use the bathroom, but you can't get rid of your worries right before bed. Or perhaps you're now confident that, no matter what goofy thoughts OCD puts in your head, you're not going to hurt anyone—except your baby sister. When you're looking at the tasks left to accomplish, it's important to group them in some way. What makes them different from the ones you've already accomplished? Talk about why they're at the top of your list and still seem pretty scary.

Also talk about what you've learned from using your toolkit, talking back to OCD, and breaking OCD's rules. Over the last month you honed a lot of tools. You may have started using certain tools or methods so instinctively that you could almost forget how useful they've become. Think about it now. What did you use most? What really came through for you when you were in a tight spot and needed help fast? What was the most comforting when the fear thermometer really started to heat up? Who has been the most helpful and the least judgmental? It may not be the person you expect—someone in the background, that in your memories of your last month might have been on the edge of your life, maybe someone you'd see out of the corner of your mind's eye. Gather these people and those tools together now. They're your most faithful allies, your most reliable tools. Make sure you use them to their fullest in the coming weeks.

Start Advanced Tasks

There's no denying that the level of resisting OCD you're about to do seems more difficult. But you have a long résumé of successes to remind you that you can do it and it really isn't harder, since none of it makes any sense. The best way to reinforce that idea is to take the plunge. Pick a difficult task for the coming week, maybe one that you've listed as a 5 or a 6 on your fear thermometer. Go to the very top of the work zone, where you're winning some of the time but not easily. You know that when you've done tough tasks in the past, your fear thermometer has gone up to an 8, and you've handled it by talking back to OCD, using chill-out methods, doing something fun, and finding creative ways to break OCD's rules. So pick something that will be a challenge.

Keep in mind as you work on it, though, that you will have achieved a huge success if you simply eliminate this one task from your list after a week—or even two. You've raised the bar, and it just won't be as easy to get over it as it was when your tasks required only baby steps. Maybe you'll need to break this one up into baby steps, too, with the goal of being willing to expose yourself to the situation and being able to avoid doing any rituals after 7-10 days of ramping up EX/RP. Keep reminding yourself that conquering one piece of OCD's territory this week is as big a success (even bigger, truly) as it was to conquer three that were ranked lower on your fear thermometer.

Every time you conquer one such task, tackle another, but make sure you stay with each task for at least a week, doing daily homework until the trigger no longer makes you uncomfortable when you encounter it and don't do OCD's rituals. Remind yourself that thinking of OCD as hard is just part of OCD's tricks—they are all easy if you keep perspective. Keep going until you've checked off the last item on your symptom list.

You know how to do it, which is why we've summed up such a big assignment in such a few words. Now it's up to you, but always remember those who are there to help you.

Give Your Parents Permission to Stop Participating in Rituals

During Step 6, you tried letting your parents back off from their involvement in your rituals. If it went well, now is the time to give them more freedom to do that. Let them choose some rituals to stop participating in, but remember that you still have a say. Proceed at whatever pace you're comfortable with. If you can handle letting your parents back out of all lock checking or extra laundry or counting rituals, go ahead. But if you know you can deal with only a slower pace, the goal is to negotiate what seems acceptable to all of you. You shouldn't be pushed into trying anything that will set you back because it's too hard, but your parents will want to ensure that progress is in fact made.

As you did on a preliminary basis in Step 6, you should all brainstorm to anticipate problems that will come up and how you can handle them. Your parents will balance refusing to cooperate with rituals with giving you additional support to help you manage distress.

Keep going! Four to six weeks can seem like a long time, but when it's over, so is OCD!

Taking Stock

Use the OCD scale to check how you're doing and add the ratings to your graph. By now you should have a graph that looks a lot like this, assuming 12 weeks for the whole program:

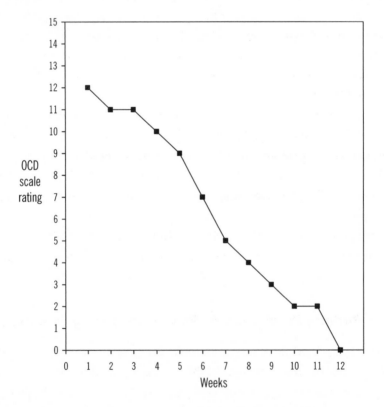

Keep in mind, though, that Steps 6 and 7 may take 10-12 weeks, so if you aren't done, that's OK. Just keep at it so long as progress is steady. If you've had OCD for a long time, you may be very happy to be at this point; you may feel like slowing down now and doing other things instead. We don't encourage this—why quit when you're ahead and you can send OCD packing for good? But you won't wipe out all your previous success whatever you do. Talk to your parents and/or therapist about where you want to go from here.

Step 7: Instructions for Parents

Get Ready

At this point in the program it's somewhat natural for your child's progress to slow. He may think that this means he's doing something wrong or the program isn't working for him anymore. Be prepared to assure him that that's not the case and point to how many symptoms he's eliminated from the chart and how few are left to tackle. This means that your child's territory probably has grown a lot bigger as OCD's has gotten a lot smaller. Take every opportunity to remind him of that.

If your child is discouraged by slower progress made during Step 6, review the suggestions in this chapter for dealing with plateaus.

Move Onward and Upward

At this point in the program kids should have internalized the strategy of exposure and response prevention. This means that they are so accustomed to using it that they often start applying it to actions, situations, and triggers that they haven't specifically chosen to work on that week. This is, of course, exactly what we want kids to achieve, namely to internalize the strategy for eliminating and even preventing OCD. It's what makes it possible for them to avoid relapsing—to squash OCD quickly and decisively if OCD ever rears its ugly head in the future. But if your child starts using EX/RP on really difficult triggers, she could inadvertently try to tackle targets that are still beyond her ability. This will result in failure and discouragement. Plateauing could be one sign that your child is experiencing this kind of problem. Be sure to talk to your child about any attempts to do EX/RP on unplanned targets. Some kids don't even consciously think about what they've been doing and need help in bringing these EX/RP failures to the surface.

If your child is attacking unplanned targets and failing, be sure to remind him

that this is really hard work and that he needs to stick to the tasks you've all discussed until he gets through Step 7.

One additional tip for responding to your child's plateau is something that's
been said before in this book:

Practice kindness and compassion and exercise patience. Remember that OCD is an
illness and that the goal is to get as well as possible as quickly as possible. Some kids
go fast; others go more slowly. Always remember that a child who has hit a plateau
is probably much more upset by this than you are. So if you feel impatient or start to
wonder whether your child is really working hard enough to fight OCD, stop yourself before you say anything or do anything that will seem like tightening the screws
on your child. This is *not* the time to offer reminders to do the homework, no matter
how adept you've become at nudging gently. Instead just be patient, support the
idea of your child's taking a break from assigning herself new tasks, and count on
OCD to push her forward again. We've said it before—no one hates OCD as much as
your child does. By itself, that will almost always get your child going again soon.

Helping younger kids: Littler kids still will need lots and lots of help at this stage,
because the tasks they must tackle can be pretty frightening. Your belief that the
child can do it will be invaluable. Just watch out for the tendency to slip into old
forms of reassurance that are actually ways of participating in the child's rituals,
such as reassuring your child that the doors are locked, that the drinking glasses
have been washed three times, that his clothing is arranged in the closet in the order
that OCD demands, and so forth. Your reassurances should be limited to reminders
that the child has a terrific toolkit, formidable brainpower, a great sense of humor,
the courage to continue to take on OCD, and an impressive track record in beating
OCD.

To reinforce those claims, consider tacking up the maps of OCD that you've
drawn throughout the program. Also put up the graph your child has been making
based on the OCD scale completed at the end of each step. Post them where your
child can see them often, and she'll have a graphic reminder of the rate at which
OCD's territory has shrunk and her territory has grown. If that kind of reinforcement seems especially effective with your child, try other graphic depictions as well.
You could making drawings that show your child climbing a ladder, with each rung
representing an item eliminated from the symptom list. Be inventive, perhaps pair-
ing the trip up the symptom chart or task list with the rewards received and
expected.

Helping teenagers: More than younger kids, your teenager is likely to do two
things that will slow you all down. First, he may become overconfident and impatient and let EX/RP loose on all of OCD before he's ready. Naturally, he wants to be
done with OCD and get on with his life. You may have to remind him to try to take
it easy and stick with the work zone. It is what got him here. Second, he may have
had enough relief from OCD to feel like he's made enough progress and wants to go
back to listening to music or being with friends rather than doing the program. Ask
him to do his best to be honest: if he's reached a plateau, he shouldn't rush to get off

it but take stock, looking closely at whether he's pushing himself too hard and too fast or not hard enough. If he keeps going too fast, that first step off the plateau could take him a step down rather than a leap up. If he's slowed down and didn't need to, ask him if he feels ready to commit to forging ahead again. If not, ask him if he needs help exploring the reasons. If he says he can handle it on his own, ask him to let you know on an agreed-on day what he's uncovered and what his game plan is.

Some teens will get all wrapped up in the idea that the top of the symptom ladder is harder and end up making it harder than it actually is. You can remind your daughter that what OCD says isn't true—the reality is that there isn't any ladder that she has to work her way up. It is all nonsense, but it surely doesn't feel that way, which is why we suggest that kids try to stay in the work zone as much as possible. If the idea is appealing, suggest dropping the idea that not just OCD but any unwanted thought is somehow part of who we are. By part of who we are, we mean that which has anything to do with personal truth. Try to explore with your teen what it means to identify with the "you" that is watching, not telling a personal story. Once he has the idea, when OCD shows up, the practice is as follows: Relax and pay attention to what is actually happening; accept that OCD is present; *do not* identify OCD as personal in any way, even to the point of dropping any story he might hold about OCD; and just go on about his business. After a while, if he doesn't make an idol of it, OCD will just fade away. For more practice, try the same tactic with other irritations or frustrating desires: relax and pay attention to what is actually happening, acknowledge what is present, identify with the you that is watching, drop the personal part of the story, and just go on doing the best you can in that moment. Try this yourself. You might surprise yourself with how much more ease and well-being enters your life when you are not arguing with reality but just doing the best you can with whatever comes your way. If this doesn't make sense to you, don't worry about it; just stay with the program as you've been working it.

How a therapist can help: If your child needs help talking through the next level she's approaching and how she's going to tackle it, visiting the therapist or even talking things through on the phone will save her a lot of wasted time in the weeks ahead. Be sure she understands this fact so that she feels OK asking for this help.

If you think your child may be stalled because of mental rituals, delayed rituals, or some other OCD-serving recourse to avoid the discomfort of the more difficult tasks at hand, be sure to consult a therapist now. It's hard for parents to ask a child about whether he is resorting to such maneuvers without sounding critical. A therapist will know how to help your child bring these behaviors to the surface without guilt and then deal with them.

Another ingredient that may get your child stuck on a plateau is a co-occurring (comorbid) condition, such as undiagnosed ADHD. See page 46 for more information on the other psychiatric disorders that kids with OCD sometimes have. If you've explored other avenues to see why your child is stuck and still can't get him off that plateau, ask a therapist whether the child may need to be screened for another disorder.

Start Advanced Tasks

Help your child stick to one or two tasks at a time, and don't be surprised if this step takes longer than 6 weeks. If the child has six items left on her list at the beginning of Step 7, it could take 8 weeks or even more to get through them. As long as progress continues, the pace isn't so important as just making steady progress. Don't let your child get discouraged. As you remind her of how well she's doing against OCD, also remind her of what else she has going for her, and focus on the things she's been able to do now that OCD isn't around so much.

If your child balks at the beginning of this advanced EX/RP work, remind her how much she enjoys some things that are scary *because* they're scary—like roller coasters and monster movies and fireworks. If she swims, remember the trip from the shallow end to the high dive. Talk to her about the great feeling of accomplishment she gets after braving something intimidating, like trying out for the basketball team or the school play. No pain, no gain. And the gain lasts forever, while the pain is temporary and fades even from memory pretty quickly.

ALEXIS (age 4): I don't want to eat corn. It has bugs.

MOM: That's Stinky talking. If Stinky wins, you told me you won't get dessert because you know you have to eat your corn to get dessert, Stinky or no Stinky. Besides, you like corn.

ALEXIS: OK, I'll eat it. I hate Stinky.

PATRICK (age 13): I've had it with this stuff. All you do is talk about OCD. I'd rather do anything except talk about OCD.

DAD: OK, we won't talk about it so long as you can stay with the program. All we need is for you to check in so that we know that you're doing what's necessary. That'd be OK?

PATRICK: Sure, Dad, whatever.

[*Patrick set up the symptom chart and did his own EX/RP.*]

PATRICK: Dad, I need you and Mom to stop answering my questions about God. Don't ask me why; just don't answer my questions, OK?

DAD: Sure, Patrick, glad you're on top of OCD.

MARSHALL (age 17): Let's see, I have four things left, but I'd better break them down so I'm sure that they won't be too hard. How about we make four separate lists, breaking up the RP part into easy, medium, and hard? I'll go for each one over a week, and that'll do it. Now about that CD, can I have a videogame instead?

MOM: That works for me!

BILL (age 16): You know, I was really pissed off at my friend Jim today, and I tried just watching my anger and not identifying with it. It let me see Jim in a whole new way, and I wasn't so mad afterward. Then, when I went into the bathroom to do my EX/RP task, I did the same thing. No story, just watched, and it was a lot easier than I expected.

Mom: Funny you should mention it, but I tried the same tactic with Mabel—you know, the woman at work with the really obnoxious voice? Maybe there's something to learn here that goes beyond OCD?

Talk to your child's siblings about how they can help, too. By now you should know who has the patience and who your child's closest allies are among family and friends. See if you can enlist their aid in new ways or on a new level.

How a therapist can help: These weeks can be difficult to get through, even with all the support your child can muster from family and friends. If your child is working with a therapist, consider scheduling more frequent telephone check-ins than in the past. Also consider having the therapist coach your child in each new EX/RP task, at the site where the task will have to be performed, before the child launches into the work on her own.

Getting Your Child's Permission to Stop Participating in Rituals

This goal is a tricky balancing act. You need to make sure your child moves forward, but you can't insist on progress that is too rapid. If your child can't give you blanket permission to stop participating in rituals at this point, devote whatever time it takes to come up with a step-by-step strategy for withdrawing from rituals a little at a time. You may have to be strong if your child tries to back out of the "deal" when anxiety spikes, but in that case you should resort to what you know works with your child, just as your child must always resort to what works for him.

Helping younger kids: Make a game of it, with something fun at the end. No, tackling OCD isn't the same as playing Candy Land, but you can still enjoy giving OCD a hard time, with a treat at the end.

Helping teenagers: Your teenager's biggest enemy in trying to reach this goal might end up being her pride. She might feel that she *has* to give you permission to stop helping with her rituals. After all, how can she tell you to stay out of her social life or ask you to trust her to get her homework and chores done or to give her the keys to the car—or how can she decide where she's going to go to college—if she needs to have your reassurance that all the doors and windows are locked before she can turn her light out at night? A teenager needs to find a way to separate her right and need to become an independent young adult from her need to assert her independence from and mastery over OCD. They're not the same thing—not as far as your child is concerned, and not as far as you are concerned. She can ask for the keys to the car and at the same time ask you to take your withdrawal from OCD rituals slowly—as long as you do so surely, as well. Here it is important to emphasize that OCD is an illness, not good or bad behavior, and that getting rid of OCD is a key to getting out of high school, going off to college, and doing all the things that young adults like to do. There's no time like the present to get a hold of OCD and wring its neck.

How a therapist can help: If you and your child end up at loggerheads over your withdrawal from OCD rituals, call for help. It's easy to become impatient once you see how far your child has come. It's natural to reason that if your child could conquer things that he feared so strongly just a few short weeks ago, then surely he doesn't need your checking and reassurances anymore. That sounds logical, but remember that when your child works on an EX/RP task, he's in charge. When you back out of one, your child can feel as if he's given up some of that control over this fight against OCD. So even though he can stand tough against OCD all by himself in so many areas, he may still be loath to give up your participation in certain rituals. As long as you can make some progress in this area, you're doing fine. But if you find yourself unable to work at your child's pace, call in a therapist to choose tasks that, in his or her professional judgment, your child can handle and to advise you on strategies for managing your child's distress so that your child continues to trust you to be supportive in the battle against OCD.

Taking Stock

Do a reality check at this point. This is a good time to consider whether your child's motivation is truly good, whether other things are getting in the way, or whether OCD is too hard for her to use a self-help program. If things aren't going as well as we've been predicting, it's time to seriously consider involving a mental health professional, if you haven't done so. Maybe this would be a good time to think about medications if your child's progress is slow or if some other problem, such as depression or social anxiety, seems to be getting in the way of EX/RP.

7

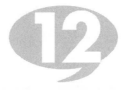

Step 8: Keeping OCD Away for Good

WHEW.

That was a lot of work, wasn't it? If you've followed the program from Step 1 all the way through Step 7, done your homework, and gotten support from your parents and help from your therapist, I probably don't have to tell you it was worth it. Take a look at your map of OCD to remind yourself just how worthwhile all that effort was. At this point OCD should be pretty much out of your life space. Here's what that might look and feel like:

I can eat lunch with my friends again. I don't have to go eat in the assistant principal's office anymore. Sometimes when I go into the cafeteria I feel like OCD is going to stop me for a second, but I just laugh and say, "Yeah, you can stay out. It's too dirty in here for you—but not for me!"

—Maggie, age 9

Some of the guys used to look at me like I was weird or something, but you know what? I don't act weird anymore, so they'll get used to the real me pretty soon.

—Zach, age 14

Mommy says I'm the toughest kid she knows. But she says I don't have to be too brave—if OCD ever tries to come back, all I have to do is tell her and she'll help me.

—Dustin, age 6

I can't believe it. I'm going to college. And I'm pretty sure it'll be OK. I won't miss classes because I'm busy hoarding my books and papers, and

I'll probably turn in my papers on time—at least about as on time as any other freshman! There's a great counseling center at my school, and I'll check in with them if I have any problems.

—Tanisha, age 18

I don't know. Everything's going great right now, but I have this feeling sometimes that old Nasty is hanging around, just waiting for me to get lazy or something. I hope he won't come back. . . .

—Brianna, age 11

You know, a lot of what I learned in confronting OCD, I somehow seem to be able to apply to other stuff. If you just deal with it, life isn't so hard.

—Alan, age 14

If you're one of the lucky kids who feel confident they've gotten rid of OCD for good, congratulations! But if you have a few doubts, like Brianna, don't worry. Step 8 is all about preparing yourself to keep OCD away even if it tries to find its way back into your life.

The Game Plan for Step 8

After reviewing what you accomplished in Step 7, do the reading and other preparation listed under "Get Ready" and then follow the instructions for Step 8. There's no time limit here, though I generally allow a week or two for this step with most kids. This is your leap back into the rest of your terrific life!

Remember that you have now learned all the skills that you need to deal with OCD. At the first hint that OCD is trying to return, you can always pull out the strategies you've learned in this book. Also remember, *never hesitate to ask for help*.

One more time, put up the "Getting Stronger Every Day" chart. Once you've checked off all the days that you keep up the good fight against OCD, you'll have a nice thick collection of evidence of your hard work.

Get Ready—or Look Back . . . to Look Forward

I'm not going to ask you to train a magnifying glass on the work you did over the last several weeks in Step 7. Instead, I want you to take a few minutes to rate yourself on the OCD scale again. How did you do? A 1-3 is terrific—a home run. A 4-6 is very good—OCD is around, and you need to keep at it, but it's not bugging you much at all. If you started way higher on the scale, this is a home run, too. If you have any doubts about your perception of yourself, ask one of your parents and/or your therapist to rate you on these scales, too. If they have the same general view of where you stand and how far you've come that you do, you'll know you're seeing yourself clearly. You'll be ready to graduate with just a little more effort at this step.

If your ratings on the scale are lower, or if those reported by your parent or therapist are lower than yours, go back to your symptom chart and see where the trouble lies. Then work on the remaining bothersome hiccups for another week and complete the scale again.

There's no summary chart for this step for you to post, but many kids find it helpful to remind themselves of what they've accomplished, so they tape up the Taking Stock graph.

How do you get ready for the rest of your life? Sounds like a pretty big question, and we'll bet, in fact, you do have big plans and big dreams. With OCD out of the way, there's no reason you can't make them all happen. Getting ready for the rest of your life as far as this program is concerned, however, means being prepared for little slips and lapses to occur, *even if OCD seems to have vanished completely at this moment*. That's just the way this illness is. Occasionally, when you least expect it, one of the old worries or upsetting thoughts might pop into your mind. Or maybe one of the flavors of OCD that you've never had will show up someday. When that happens, it doesn't mean that all your work has been for nothing. It doesn't mean OCD has taken over your territory again or that it's here to stay (any more than getting the hiccups again means you're stuck with them). It doesn't mean you have to start all over with Step 1. It does mean that it's time to haul out your toolkit and put it to work right away. It does mean that you might want to tell your parents or therapist that OCD showed up uninvited again. When you have a slip or lapse, as many kids do, just show OCD the door immediately. Relax, remember that you know what OCD is, accept that it is present, and apply your toolkit, especially EX/RP, and that'll be the end of it. Most important, let OCD know it's not wanted and not welcome. Don't let it get started because you don't want to admit that it's shown up again. Take quick action and it will slink off into the background again, and you can get back to your plans and dreams.

Get Going

Make Saying No to OCD Second Nature

The experience other doctors and I have had with adults and kids at our clinic has shown that the key to keeping OCD at bay is bossing it back so automatically that you hardly have to think about it. Put differently, when the stop signal is working again, when an OCD hiccup starts up, the brain will automatically try to turn it off instead of letting it run. You may need to help a bit, though. Mostly you'll just do it because you know how, and the OCD hiccups will go away, and you'll never give it a second thought. That's what we want you to learn to do with the occasional unannounced appearance of OCD.

Start by imagining that OCD really wants to make a comeback. Where do you think it would show up? Maybe as a hiccup that you had a lot of trouble with during the program? As one that made your fear thermometer go pretty high? In an area that you encounter all the time?

Maggie's main symptom area was places where food is eaten, so she had lots of trouble with OCD—which she called Piggy—when she was at restaurants, especially ones with lots of "sloppy" kids at them, and the school cafeteria. She thought OCD might be most likely to pop up when she went to a new fast-food place for the first time.

OCD mainly told Zach he had to tap doors he went through a certain number of times, tap the walls in long hallways, or tap the floor in rooms he hadn't been in before. He thought OCD might show up sometime next year, when he started high school and the whole building was new.

Dustin thought OCD might try to come back when he was at his grandma's house for Thanksgiving and had to wash his hands before dinner. He felt pretty sure of himself at his own house but wasn't sure it would be as easy to resist washing over and over at Grandma's house.

Tanisha thought OCD might try to bug her if she was ever rushing to finish a paper on time once she started college, because being nervous reminds her of how OCD used to make her feel.

Brianna had a hard time imagining where OCD might pop up; thinking about it scared her at first because she thought her therapist was saying she hadn't really done well in getting rid of OCD and that things would never really be better. Her parents and her therapist cleared up that idea and helped her make her toolkit sort of like an extra hand—there to assist when she needed it, but so much a part of her that she hardly noticed when she was using it.

Once you've decided where OCD is likely to try to worm its way back into your life, imagine what would happen, letting yourself picture the incident in living color with all its details. Every 1 to 2 minutes while you imagine this, use your fear thermometer to rate how you're feeling. Use everything in your toolkit to get through this imagined foray by OCD, especially all the positive pep talk you learned to give yourself during Step 3 (Chapter 7). Keep it up till the fear thermometer reads "zero."

Brianna ultimately decided that OCD was likely to come back someday when she was about to touch an unfamiliar doorknob. Maybe she'd be walking down the hallway a few years from now in her high school, go to reach for the doorknob to a classroom, and all of a sudden she'd be terrified that if she touched the doorknob and then her mouth, she'd get AIDS and then spread it to her whole family, and they'd all die.

When she imagined this scene in vivid detail, her fear thermometer went up to a 7, and she started breathing heavily and really feeling panicky, as if the whole scene were real. Then she remembered what she'd learned weeks ago and had been using to brush OCD aside ever since: "Hey, Nasty," she said in her head, "you're in my way and I don't have time for this." Then she pictured herself grabbing the doorknob, then touching her mouth right away and saying "No one's going to get sick—that's just one of Nasty's lies." Finally, she imagined she'd walk into the classroom, sit down, and think about what a beautiful day it was and what she was going to do after school. This brought her fear thermometer down to zero, and she heaved a sigh of relief.

Brianna repeated this imagined scene for about half an hour and then did the same practice for each general area or "flavor" that she had listed on her symptom chart: washing, checking, repeating/arranging/counting, religious or moral scrupulosity, and hoarding. Each time, she brought in the tools from her toolkit to help her get through the encounter with OCD, but she always started with acknowledging OCD with a simple "Hey, Nasty" or "Hi, Nasty" to instantly remind herself that this was OCD talking, not sensible Brianna. She also reminded herself of the important guidelines that make the whole program work and should be used anytime OCD tries to come back:

1. You are normal, not "crazy."
2. OCD is a brain illness, not good or bad behavior.
3. All family members deserve deep respect. You, the person who is ill, deserve sympathy and kindness.
4. Relax, name OCD as OCD, and observe it as though you're watching a TV program.
5. Remind yourself that OCD hiccups are not your thoughts, that they make no sense; then believe it.
6. Make a map of OCD, ranking triggers, obsessions, and rituals from easy to hard to resist.
7. Identify the work zone, where you already resist successfully more than 50% of the time.

8. Using EX/RP, convert OCD symptoms in the work zone to 100% success until OCD is gone.

9. Be patient and kind as you move up to harder stuff—it'll be easier when you get there.

10. OCD is bad for your brain and your life—commit yourself to following the program!

You might do this rehearsing for about a week, or two if it makes you feel stronger, imagining OCD attempts in several different areas for a few minutes a day—just long enough to get the fear thermometer up a bit and let it come back down. Because these aren't real OCD hiccups, it doesn't take much time. It's more like scouting ahead to make sure that you know what to do.

For teenagers: The biggest danger for you, in my experience, may be letting your pride take over. Kids who've successfully ousted OCD are rightfully proud of what they've accomplished and understandably relieved to put it all behind them. But ignorance isn't bliss in this case. If you notice OCD coming back, don't pretend it isn't happening, try not to be overconfident that you can just ignore it without using your toolkit, and try not to let pride stand in the way of your talking to your parents or your therapist about it. The sooner you take action against OCD, the faster the slip will become a thing of the past.

Celebrate Your Graduation!

Wow, you've come a long way! Completing this program gives you a lot to be proud of: You've taken a stand and run OCD out of your life. You've relearned how much you have going for you once you're not preoccupied with OCD all the time. You've given yourself the chance to start dreaming about and planning all the great things life has in store for you. You've been brave and tough and smart. You deserve a celebration!

Deciding how to celebrate your graduation from this program should be a family affair. Everyone has been affected by OCD, and now everyone has played a positive role in showing OCD the door. Ideally, your graduation ceremony should be something the whole family will enjoy. Let your imaginations run wild and do what you'd do to celebrate any other important graduation, award, or stellar achievement. Just make sure these elements are included:

• You should get a certificate marking this achievement. It always helps to have an acknowledgment of all your work that you can see and feel. Your parents

If You're Going Off Your Medication . . .

For kids who have been taking medication while working through this program, sometime after the completion of Step 8 the therapist and prescribing doctor are likely to recommend stopping the medicine. (This will be done gradually over time, and it's hard to say exactly when your doctors will want to do this, but you should be prepared for this eventuality.) If this applies to you, there are two things you should know:

1. *Remember that it's not the medicine that has kept OCD away but your own efforts.* I like to think of medications as like water wings or training wheels on a bike. They help you while you're learning to swim, but unless you acquire the skills needed to keep your head above water, the water wings won't protect you once you take them off. As discussed in Chapter 4, our long-term research study showed that the combination of this program and medication was the most effective treatment, especially for kids with more severe OCD. But we believe it's the program you've just completed that's the critical ingredient, and other scientists' research has confirmed this, too, showing that the great majority of people with OCD relapse once medication is withdrawn if they haven't also gone through a CBT program like this one. Another study showed that when people who were taking medication were instructed *not* to do the opposite of what OCD tells them, as you've learned to do in this program, all the positive benefits they had gotten from medication disappeared. This means it looks like the EX/RP work you've been doing throughout this book is necessary to make medication work, not the other way around! Keep this in mind when your doctor says it's time to cut you loose from medication. You're not going to lose everything you've gained when you stop taking those pills—not as long as you hold on to that toolkit you've worked so hard to build!

2. *A booster session with the therapist can help you make sure your toolkit is tough enough.* Some kids understandably get a little nervous about what will happen when the medication is stopped. Even if they know they have a great toolkit, somewhere in the back of their minds they can't help wondering whether they'll notice a difference in their ability to resist OCD when they're first off the medicine. That's why it's a good idea to go see your therapist for a refresher session. During that session your therapist can go over all your strategies, helping you dust off and polish any you feel are a little rusty and providing you with the reassurance you deserve that you can resist OCD on your own. Think of it as going back for a refresher swimming lesson. You know you've learned to swim, but just in case you have any doubts before you throw those water wings away, you can get a little help from the experts in making sure your skills are as good as they can be.

can work one up using a computer and some of the special paper that's available at office supply stores or just their computer tools. Or you can fill in your name on my letter to you at the end of this chapter and pull that out of the book. Make it part of your "closing ceremony" and hang it somewhere in your room to remind yourself of what you've achieved—or where everyone in your family can see it too if you want.

• The celebration should be essentially a bragging session, where everyone tells stories about all the ways you've gotten rid of OCD and all the things you are now free to do that were impossible when OCD stood in the way.

• The possibility that OCD will try to come back should always be acknowledged out loud, but at the same time, remind yourselves of your hard-earned ability to face these encounters with OCD and still emerge victorious.

• Other people should be notified of your success, to make it all the more real and to put it on a par with other grand achievements, such as a school graduation or an athletic championship.

A Letter to You from Dr. March

To my friend _____,

    Though we don't know each other, you are the real reason I wrote this book, and I am very happy to see how well you've done. When I began working with kids with OCD in the 1980s, most of my doctor colleagues said that kids with OCD were untreatable. Well, it is a good thing I listened to my patients and their parents, who were convinced, as I was, that we could make CBT work for kids with OCD. I wasn't about to accept anything else, and neither were my patients—and now that includes you and your family, too. Every week I receive a few e-mails from children and parents around the world thanking me for making CBT available to them. But I'm not the one who deserves the gratitude. It is you and all the other kids who hate OCD enough to want to get better who've made this possible. It is you who've taught me how to make the OCD hiccups stop. Congratulations to you and to your family—you are really terrific.

    Take care and be well,

    John

Getting Stronger Every Day . . . Step 8

At the end of each day, check off whether you've followed the instructions for Step 8, making talking back to OCD second nature so you can pick up your toolkit again at a moment's notice whenever you need it. This final form includes 2 weeks' worth of days, but you may need only a week.

Day 71 ☐ I did the homework for Step 8.

Day 72 ☐ I did the homework for Step 8.

Day 73 ☐ I did the homework for Step 8.

Day 74 ☐ I did the homework for Step 8.

Day 75 ☐ I did the homework for Step 8.

Day 76 ☐ I did the homework for Step 8.

Day 77 ☐ I did the homework for Step 8.

Day 78 ☐ I did the homework for Step 8.

Day 79 ☐ I did the homework for Step 8.

Day 80 ☐ I did the homework for Step 8.

Day 81 ☐ I did the homework for Step 8.

Day 82 ☐ I did the homework for Step 8.

Day 83 ☐ I did the homework for Step 8.

Day 84 ☐ I did the homework for Step 8.

Step 8: Instructions for Parents

YOU MAY NOT BELIEVE you've come this far. But if your child has stuck with this program all the way through, life is probably back where it should be, or at least pretty close. This chapter gives you a few ideas for keeping it that way.

Get Going

Make Saying No to OCD Second Nature

Your job is threefold in helping to prevent little slips and minor attempts at a comeback by OCD from turning into a real relapse:

1. Remind your child that a relapse really is unlikely, because she has a terrific toolkit to draw on, and with a little extra practice to turn the tools into the equivalent of extra hands, the child can call the toolkit into service at a moment's notice, meaning that OCD can be shooed away in the blink of an eye. At first you might want to offer these reminders spontaneously and regularly, though you'll have to gauge their value by the reaction you get from your son or daughter. If your child starts rolling his eyes or saying "I know, I KNOW" when you start your pep talk, you know you're overdoing it. After a week or two, if things continue to go well, you can probably offer these reminders only when your child expresses some kind of doubt or worry about OCD's really having gone away.

2. Help your child be alert to the signs that OCD is trying to make a comeback. At this point in the program, you might say something like this:

"You've been watching your mind long enough to know that weird fears and odd thoughts are common. Mostly, they just show up and go away, but if they stick around even when you don't want them to and they fall into one of the typical flavors of OCD, hey, you may be experiencing a sneak attack of OCD. The temptation is to take the hiccup seriously for two reasons: First, who wants to admit to himself that OCD is back? Second, it may on the surface seem reasonable—it is helpful if this isn't the case, but it often is. The key is to relax, ask whether this is OCD, and if you think it is, put your toolkit to work before it has a chance to mushroom out of control. I'll be here to help if you need me." Be matter-of-fact but unfailingly kind.

Also, watch out for the tendency to hover over your child, watching over her like a hawk, ready to dive in at the slightest hint of a relapse. This kind of overvigilance can have a rebound effect, making your child so nervous that she'll feel the same way she felt when OCD was constantly "supervising."

3. If you've encouraged the child to use her toolkit but OCD seems to be gaining a foothold anyway, don't waste any time in scheduling a "booster" session with her therapist. The best way to ensure that a lapse doesn't turn into a relapse is to act fast. A booster session with the therapist might reveal that the child has forgotten some critical element in the strategies for resisting OCD or that the child just needs some additional practice in using the toolkit, which can be initiated and guided by the therapist but conducted at home.

How a therapist can help: If you're not sure where OCD is likely to find a chink in your child's armor first, schedule a session with the therapist so your child can talk it over with the therapist and start his practice in keeping OCD at bay. Brianna needed a little reassurance that she really had succeeded in this program and had taken her life back from OCD. Once she got that, both from her parents and from her therapist, she found it easier to think about where OCD might attack first; but she got a little nervous again when she started going through her whole symptom list, so it was easier for her to do this part of Step 8 with her therapist. She checked in with the therapist once a week for the next 3 weeks and reported on how she did with her imagined encounters with OCD, from notes she kept about her fear thermometer readings in her notebook. At the end of that time, her therapist pronounced her ready to graduate, and she and her family had a celebration unlike any other before.

Another way that the therapist can help is with kids who have been taking medication and are about to stop. Some kids—see the box on page 247—give those little pills a lot more credit than they deserve for keeping OCD away. The therapist, in a booster session scheduled to coincide with discontinuing medication, can reassure the child that the medication was there only to help him get the most out of the program he just completed. At the same time, the booster session can reinforce the child's skill in using the strategies so that they provide enduring protection against OCD.

Celebrate Your Child's Graduation!

How much you choreograph the whole graduation ceremony and celebration will depend on your child's wishes and maturity. Shy kids might want a low-key dinner with just the immediate family and may not want to announce their victory over

OCD to a whole spectrum of other people, because they may never have felt comfortable talking about their illness to begin with. Encourage those kids to pick at least one person—a close friend or an extended family member who's already aware of the problem, at least to some degree—to notify of their accomplishments. Telling someone else has a way of solidifying the success in the child's mind. Saying it out loud makes it real, and getting the typical congratulatory response reinforces what a big achievement it really is.

A more outgoing child may want to plan the whole affair as though it's the event of the year, and you should let that happen to the extent that you can, within reason and your means.

There are a million different ways to acknowledge what this graduation means to the child's life. To prepare for your bragging session, you could add to the child's graduation certificate a scroll on which you've written a long list of things the child can now do that OCD prohibited. For Brianna, whose obsessions centered on contamination fears, the list could include everything from swimming in the community pool (and using the shower) to going to a movie (because she'd now be able to risk having to use the public restroom) to sleeping later on schooldays (because no extra time needs to be allotted for washing up before breakfast) to shaking hands with new acquaintances to sleeping over at a friend's house to joining the soccer team.

Tailor the celebration to your unique family and child. Most kids won't want to do much. Teens will want to do it with friends without parents and without OCD mentioned.

A final word: Remember, you've accomplished an awful lot along with your child. You've developed a whole new attitude toward OCD that was critical to your child's success in talking back and getting rid of the symptoms that were interfering in the child's life and yours. If you've followed the guidelines in this program, you may very well have a stronger bond with your child than ever before. What you've learned with OCD can translate into other areas of your life if you let it. The world is filled with challenges, inside and out. A little kindness, paying close attention, not making idols of what we want or don't want, and doing whatever we can to make things at least a little better isn't a bad formula for happiness.

For additional information on any subject not covered in this book, see the Resources at the back. And never hesitate to contact a therapist for help, now or in the future.

8

Summaries of the Steps

STEP 1: What Kind of Treatment Is This, Anyway?

- Spend Week 1 on this step, and if things are going well, add in Step 2 at some point during this week. Check off that you've done the following homework on the form at the end of Chapter 5.

Gather Your Team

- Get used to the idea that you're in charge of how you "talk to" OCD and that everyone else is there to support and cheer as needed, including your parents, teachers, and other adults in your life.
- Make sure you have a therapist if you need one.

Get a Picture of the Whole Program

- Read Part I, have your parents explain the eight steps, or talk it all over with your therapist.

Give OCD a Funny Nickname or Learn to Call It by Its Medical Name

- It's not you that's coming up with these funny ideas and rituals; it's OCD. All week, call it what it is—an illness separate from you.

Start Noticing Where OCD Wins and Where You Win

- Pay attention to where you can already resist what OCD tells you—it's not in charge of as much of your life as you think!
- Fill out the Taking Stock scale and plot the number on the graph.

253

STEP 2: Talking Back to OCD

- Spend about a week (maybe part of Week 1 and part of Week 2) on this step, adding in Steps 3 and 4 sometime before the end of Week 2. Check off that you've done the following homework for 30–60 minutes a day on the form at the end of Chapter 5.

Make OCD the Problem

- Think about and talk over the questions that help you see OCD as an illness.

Start to Map OCD

- Take a close look over the week at the obsessions and compulsions that bug you and then list five to eight symptoms on your chart. Add any symptoms you notice during the week.

Get to Know the Fear Thermometer

- Give the symptoms on your chart a fear "temperature." Add the temperature to your chart whenever you add a symptom.
- Fill out the Taking Stock scale and plot the number on the graph.

STEP 3: Making a Map

- Spend about a week on this step, adding in Step 4 sometime before the end of Week 2. Check off that you've done the following homework for 30–60 minutes a day on the form at the end of Chapter 5.

Brainpower: A New Way of Thinking about OCD

- Learn and practice four ways of showing yourself how little sense it makes to listen to OCD:

    1. Keep bossing back OCD to scout it out.
    2. Give yourself a pep talk.
    3. Cut OCD down to size.
    4. Let OCD float by.

- Test out the brainpower techniques throughout the week and write down, in order, the ones that work best for you. You might even write a little "script" for how you'll talk back to OCD when caught by surprise.

Complete Your Map of OCD

- Review your symptom chart and during this week observe OCD and make changes and additions until your chart lists all the symptoms you have to deal with.

Reward Yourself for Progress Made

- Give yourself a pat on the back every time you talk back to OCD and ask your parents to set up a reward system for specific accomplishments.
- Fill out the Taking Stock scale and plot the number on the graph.

STEP 4: Finishing My Toolkit

- Spend about 4–7 days on this step. You should finish Steps 1–4 by the end of Week 2. Check off that you've done the following homework for 30–60 minutes a day on the form at the end of Chapter 5.

Fill In the Work Zone

- Figure out which symptoms and tasks fall into the work zone—fear temperatures of no more than 3.

Complete the Toolkit

- This is just a review: make sure you're comfortable using the brainpower strategies, the symptom chart with defined work zone, the fear thermometer, and the reward system before you try tackling a specific task.

Practice a Trial EX/RP Task

- Pick one symptom or task from the work zone and resist doing the rituals while in that situation. Practice over the week.
- Fill out the Taking Stock scale and plot the number on the graph.

STEP 5: Beginning to Resist

- Spend about 3 weeks on this step. Check off that you've done the following homework for 30–60 minutes a day on the form at the end of Chapter 9.

Figure Out Where Family Members and Others Get Tangled Up in OCD

- Figure out where other people get involved in OCD rituals and add these symptoms to your chart.

Choose New Symptoms to Work On

- Pick one or two relatively easy tasks from the work zone and practice resisting OCD there for 30–60 minutes a day. When you can get the fear temperature down to 0 (or at least 1, to the point where any minor discomfort doesn't get in the way of your going about your business) for 2 days in a row, you've moved that symptom into your territory. Congratulations! After doing this for 2 weeks, if you've done this with both new tasks, pick another one or two.

Learn to Break OCD's Rules

- If a task is too hard at first, break it down: delay the ritual, shorten it, do it differently, or do it slowly. In short, do it differently than OCD says.
- Learn and use the chill-out strategies for hanging in there when you feel uncomfortable: deep breathing and relaxation.

Become a Scientist Yourself

- Notice what happens during EX/RP and figure out how you can beat OCD in places that have been too hard to do it.
- Fill out the Taking Stock scale and plot the number on the graph.

STEP 6: I'm in Charge Now

- Spend about 4–6 weeks on this step. Check off that you've done the following homework for 30–60 minutes a day on the forms at the end of Chapters 9 and 10.

Set Up Rewards, Notifications, and Ceremonies to Celebrate Success

- This is a little more formal than the reward system you set up before, because now you're making bigger leaps forward. Figure out how to make your accomplishments solidly real with rewards, announcements to important people in your life, and parties or other gatherings.

Start Intermediate Tasks

- Pick a few more tasks to tackle from the work zone and practice resisting. Review at the beginning of each week and see what you can cross off your symptom chart, anything you may need to add, and fear temperatures you can change. Choose new tasks whenever you've conquered old ones. Ask your parents to start backing away from "helping" with rituals.

Consider Letting Your Parents Select a Situation for a Task

- Take this slowly and don't try it at all until you've done 4 weeks of this step—unless you're really zooming through your symptom chart.
- Fill out the Taking Stock scale and plot the number on the graph.

STEP 7: Eliminating OCD Everywhere

- Spend about 6 weeks or longer on this step, until you've crossed everything off your symptom chart. Check off that you've done the following homework for 30–60 minutes a day on the form at the end of Chapter 10.

Move Onward and Upward

- Figure out how to get off any plateau you've hit and review what (and who) has been most helpful in talking back to OCD so far.

Start Advanced Tasks

- Start with a tough task near the top of the work zone and have at it. Be patient; you might need a week to finish each task at this stage.
- Remember that the whole idea of a symptom rank is just OCD. Don't make it harder than it needs to be.

Give Your Parents Permission to Stop Participating in Rituals

- If your test run of disentangling your parents from rituals went OK, ask them to stay out of OCD for real now, but brainstorm about how they can best help you deal with OCD.
- Fill out the Taking Stock scale and plot the number on the graph.

STEP 8: Keeping OCD Away for Good

- Spend a week or two this step. The goal is to prepare yourself to react with your tools and skills if you ever see OCD trying to pop up again. Check off that you've done the following homework for 30–60 minutes a day on the form at the end of Chapter 12.

Make Saying No to OCD Second Nature

- Imagine where and how OCD might arise again, come up with a game plan, and do a little practice in your imagination.

Celebrate Your Graduation!

- Make sure you get a certificate and have some kind of party, knowing that if OCD ever tries to emerge from the background, you're prepared.

How to Find a Therapist

A therapist trained in CBT almost certainly will be more helpful to a child or teenager with OCD than one who isn't, whether you're using the program in this book or not. More and more therapists are learning about CBT and about programs such as ours, but it still might be a challenge to find one in your area who has experience in treating kids and teens with OCD.

Finding a CBT therapist can be done in three easy steps. If you still can't find a trained CBT therapist, use the same process to find a therapist you like and find out if he or she is willing to follow the program outlined in this book and in our book for therapists.

- **Step 1: Put together a list of all the CBT therapists you can find in your area.** Go to one of the following websites and use the referral tool to help locate a CBT therapist. Most of the listed CBT therapists will be doctoral or master's-level psychologists and will not do medication management. A few may be social workers or licensed professional counselors. Additional websites that have a referral service or directory are included in the Resources, but these four are good places to start within the United States:

    1. Obsessive Compulsive Foundation: *www.ocfoundation.org*
    2. Association for Behavioral and Cognitive Therapies: *www.aabt.org*
    3. Academy of Cognitive Therapy: *www.academyofct.org*
    4. Anxiety Disorders Association of America: *www.adaa.org*

Many child and adolescent psychiatrists are also now being trained in CBT for OCD. If you would like to consider medication management and CBT from a single person, consider:

American Academy of Child and Adolescent Psychiatry: *www.aacap.org*

- **Step 2: Call or e-mail each CBT therapist to see if he or she works with children or adolescents with OCD.** Here is a suggested e-mail:

Dear Dr. [therapist's name],

I am the parent of a child with OCD, and we are looking for a CBT therapist. I found your name and e-mail address through a website for [Organization]. If you are available, I would be interested in talking with you on the phone or by e-mail prior to setting up an initial appointment.

My number is [your phone number].

Thank you,

[your name]

- **Step 3: Choose a CBT therapist with whom you think you'd like to work.** Once you've made contact, you will want to ask some questions to make sure that the therapist is a good match for your child. You can ask these questions over the phone or, if you know a therapist who comes highly recommended, at an initial visit. Here are some questions you might want to ask:

  1. Can you tell me about your experience with CBT for OCD in kids? In adults?
  2. Are you familiar with John March's approach to CBT for OCD in kids? Do you use his approach or something similar?
  3. Do you work with kids and families? How might you expect to work with us as parents in helping [your child's name] recover from OCD?
  4. In your experience, about how many sessions does it take before [your child's name] might expect some progress?
  5. What are your fees? Do you take [name your insurance plan]?
  6. Would you be willing to work with [name doctor] who is managing [your child's name] medications? (if you are seeing a doctor for medications)

You'll want to be confident that the CBT therapist is a good match for you and your child. You'll want to know how he or she will conduct an evaluation and establish a treatment plan. It's very important to ask yourself how you feel about a potential therapist. Do you feel comfortable? Does he or she have the experience and knowledge you need? Without mistaking the "perfect" for the "good enough," keep looking until you're reasonably sure that you've found the doctor you need, and then get started.

- **Step 4: If you can't find a trained CBT therapist.** If you can't find a trained CBT therapist, it may be that one exists in your area, but you simply haven't found the person. Because people with OCD tend rapidly to find out who is good and who is not, you may be able to find a good therapist by contacting members of your local OCD support group. Don't be bashful about asking for advice—remember, everyone with OCD is in this boat. Use the same questions with the support group that you would use with a prospective therapist.

If you still can't find anyone, consider a "grow your own" strategy. There are many good therapists who have all the skills needed to do CBT but who for one reason or another haven't been trained. Perhaps there's a CBT therapist who works well with depression or ADHD who would do fine with our treatment manual for therapists (see the Resources) plus this self-help book. It's a bigger stretch to work with a therapist who does supportive psychotherapy or play therapy, but you may be able to find one who will work with you.

Resources

Books

Obsessive–Compulsive Disorder

The focus of this book is the hands-on program that teaches kids (and parents) how to talk back to OCD so that the illness no longer rules the family's life. The following books may be helpful in providing information on topics not covered in depth here, such as school and medications.

OCD in Children and Adolescents: A Cognitive-Behavioral Treatment Manual by John S. March and Karen Mulle. Published by The Guilford Press (1998).—The professional manual that teaches therapists how to treat kids and teens with OCD using the approach in this book.

Freeing Your Child from Obsessive–Compulsive Disorder: A Powerful, Practical Program for Parents of Children and Adolescents by Tamar Chansky. Published by Crown (2000).—A broad book that describes a treatment plan based largely on the program outlined in the book for professionals.

The Boy Who Couldn't Stop Washing: The Experience and Treatment of OCD by Judith Rapoport. Published by Plume (1999).—The groundbreaking book that introduced OCD in children to much of the world.

Polly's Magic Games: A Child's View of Obsessive Compulsive Disorder by Constance H. Foster. Published by Dilligaf (1994).—A very short book that may be a helpful introduction for children.

Obsessive Compulsive Disorder: Help for Children and Adolescents by Mitzi Waltz. Published by O'Reilly (2000).—Includes information on many different treatment approaches, including a substantial section on medication, as well as practical information on such subjects as insurance coverage and schooling.

Obsessive Compulsive Disorder: New Help for the Family by Herbert L. Gravitz. Published by Partners Publishing Group (1998).—Focuses on the effects on the family when a member (not necessarily a child) has OCD.

What to Do When Your Child Has OCD: Strategies and Solutions by Aureen Pinto Wagner. Published by Lighthouse Press (2002).—Covers a range of topics, including medications and school, in addition to the author's own CBT program.

Up and Down the Worry Hill: A Children's Book about Obsessive–Compulsive Disorder and Its Treatment by Aureen Pinto Wagner. Published by Lighthouse Press (2000).—The companion volume for kids ages 4–8 that tells a hopeful story of a child with OCD.

OCD in Adults

Older teens and parents may find it helpful to read these books about OCD in adults. Parents who have OCD may also find them helpful.

Overcoming Obsessive Compulsive Disorder: A Self-Help Guide Using Cognitive Behavioral Techniques by David Veale and Robert Willson. Published by Constable & Robinson (2005).
Stop Obsessing! by Edna B. Foa and Reid Wilson. Published by Bantam Doubleday Dell (2001).
Over and Over Again: Understanding OCD by Fugen Neziroglu and Jose A. Yaryura Tobias. Published by Jossey-Bass (1997).
Getting Control: Overcoming Your Obsessions and Compulsions by Lee Baer. Published by Plume (revised edition 2000).
Obsessive Compulsive Disorders: A Complete Guide to Getting Well and Staying Well by Fred Penzel. Published by Oxford University Press (2000).
The Doubting Disease: Help for Scrupulosity and Religious Compulsions by Joseph W Ciarrochi. Published by Paulist Press (1995).
Brain Lock: Free Yourself from Obsessive–Compulsive Behavior by Jeffrey M. Schwartz. Published by HarperCollins (1997).
The Imp of the Mind by Lee Baer. Published by Plume (2002).

Disorders Related to OCD

Feeling Good about the Way You Look: A Program for Overcoming Body Image Problems by Sabine Wilhelm. Published by The Guilford Press (2006).
The Broken Mirror: Understanding and Treating Body Dysmorphic Disorder by Katharine A. Phillips. Published by Oxford University Press (2005).
The Hair-Pulling Problem: A Complete Guide to Trichotillomania by Frederick Penzel. Published by Oxford University Press (2003).

Anxiety Disorders in Children and Adolescents

Calming Your Anxious Mind: How Mindfulness and Compassion Can Free You from Anxiety, Fear, and Panic by Jeffrey Brantley. Published by New Harbinger (2005).
Helping Your Anxious Child: A Step-by-Step Guide for Parents by Ronald M. Rapee, Susan H. Spense, Vanessa Cobham, and Ann Wignall. Published by New Harbinger (2000).
Treating Anxious Children and Adolescents: An Evidence-Based Approach by Ronald M. Rapee, Ann Wignall, Jennifer L. Hudson, and Carolyn A. Schniering. Published by New Harbinger (2000).
Help for Worried Kids: How Your Child Can Conquer Anxiety and Fear by Cynthia G. Last. Published by The Guilford Press (2006).
Worried No More: Help and Hope for Anxious Children by Aureen Pinto Wagner. Published by Lighthouse Press (2002).

Depression

Feeling Good: The New Mood Therapy by David Burns. Published by Penguin (1980).
The Feeling Good Handbook by David Burns. Published by Penguin (1999).
Treatment for Adolescents with Depression Study (TADS) Cognitive Behavior Therapy Manual. Available at *trialweb.dcri.duke.edu/tads/manuals.html*.

Internet Resources

There is a lot of very good information on the Internet, and there is also a lot of material that is inaccurate, misleading, or even harmful. Here are a few websites that have well-deserved reputations for excellence.

Professional Organizations

Association for Behavioral and Cognitive Therapies
www.aabt.org
   A good site for a referral to a therapist.

Academy of Cognitive Therapy
www.academyofct.org
   Referrals to certified cognitive therapists.

British Association for Behavioural and Cognitive Psychotherapies
www.babcp.com
   Referrals to private accredited therapists in the United Kingdom.

American Academy of Child and Adolescent Psychiatry
www.aacap.org
   Up-to-date information on issues in child psychiatry and psychiatric medications prescribed for children and teenagers; referrals to child psychiatrists; information on psychotherapy for families.

American Psychiatric Association
www.psych.org
   Links to a wealth of resources on adult and childhood psychiatric disorders, including referrals to psychiatrists.

American Psychological Association
www.apa.org
   A wealth of news and other information, plus referrals to psychologists.

Lay-Professional Organizations

Obsessive Compulsive Foundation
www.ocfoundation.org
   Links to many resources, a directory of support groups, multimedia program "OCD in the Classroom." Features teen/young adult website Organized Chaos, with its own webzine.

OCD–United Kingdom
www.ocduk.org/index.htm
   Lists of U.K. support groups; other resources for families.

OCD Action
www.ocdaction.org.uk
   Extensive lists of U.K. support groups, international resources, information on CBT and how to get it.

The Anxiety and Depression Association of America
www.adaa.org
   Extensive resources and constantly updated lists of support groups in the 50 states plus South Africa, Canada, Mexico, and Australia; referrals to therapists.

National Alliance on Mental Illness
www.nami.org
   The nation's largest grassroots mental health organization, dedicated to advocacy, support, and education. Much information on mental health in children and numerous resources.

Tourette Syndrome Association
www.tsa-usa.org
   Resources, support, education, and advocacy. Features a section just for kids and a newsletter by and for kids.

Tourette Syndrome Foundation of Canada
www.tourette.ca
   Education, advocacy, self-help, and the promotion of research. Links to similar organizations around the world.

Tourette Syndrome Association of Australia
www.tourette.org.au
   Education, support, phone counseling, newsletter. Links to other resources, including support groups, in Australia.

Tourettes Action
www.tourettes-action.org.uk
   UK's leading charity offering support for people with TS and their families.

General Information

Duke University Program in Child Affective and Anxiety Disorders
http://www2.mc.duke.edu/pcaad/pcaad_home.htm

National Institute of Mental Health (NIMH)
www.nimh.nih.gov
   Select "Clinical Trials" under "Health & Outreach." Click on "Obsessive–Compulsive Disorder (OCD)" under "Clinical Trials" to get up-to-date information on ongoing research and research results.

Expert Consensus Guidelines for OCD
www.psychguides.com
   The full guidelines discussed in Chapter 4.

Therapist's Checklist of Obsessions and Compulsions

On the following pages is the symptom screen from the Children's Yale–Brown Obsessive Compulsive Scale (CY-BOCS), which is widely used by therapists to get a full picture of OCD in a child or teenager. You can use this list to complete your map of OCD in Chapter 7.

Children's Yale–Brown Obsessive Compulsive Scale (CY-BOCS)

CY-BOCS OBSESSIONS CHECKLIST

Current	Past	
		Contamination Obsessions
_____	_____	Concern with dirt, germs, certain illnesses (e.g., AIDS)
_____	_____	Concerns or disgust with bodily waste or secretions (e.g., urine, feces, saliva)
_____	_____	Excessive concern with enviromental contaminants (e.g., asbestos, radiation, toxic waste)
_____	_____	Excessive concern with household items (e.g., cleaners, solvents)
_____	_____	Excessive concern about animals/insects
_____	_____	Excessively bothered by sticky substances or residues
_____	_____	Concerned will get ill because of contaminant
_____	_____	Concerned will get others ill by spreading contaminant (aggressive)
_____	_____	No concern with consequences of contamination other than how it might feel
_____	_____	Other (describe): _____
		Aggressive Obsessions
_____	_____	Fear might harm self
_____	_____	Fear might harm others
_____	_____	Fear harm will come to self
_____	_____	Fear harm will come to others (maybe because of something child did or did not do)
_____	_____	Violent or horrific images
_____	_____	Fear of blurting out obscenities or insults
_____	_____	Fear of doing something else embarrassing
_____	_____	Fear will act on unwanted impulses (e.g., to stab a family member)
_____	_____	Fear will steal things
_____	_____	Fear will be responsible for something else terrible happening (e.g., fire, burglary, flood)

(cont.)

Developed by Wayne K. Goodman, MD, Lawrence H. Price, MD, Steven A. Rasmussen, MD, Mark A. Riddle, MD, and Judith L. Rapoport, MD, of the Department of Psychiatry and The Child Study Center, Yale University School of Medicine; Department of Psychiatry, Brown University School of Medicine; and Child Psychiatry Branch, National Institute of Mental Health.

Investigators interested in using this rating scale should contact Wayne Goodman, MD, at the Clinical Neuroscience Research Unit, Connecticut Mental Health Center, 34 Park Street, New Haven, CT 06508 or Mark Riddle, MD, at the Yale Child Study Center, P.O. Box 3333, New Haven, CT 06510.

_____ _____ Other (describe): _____

Sexual Obsessions

_____ _____ (Are you having any sexual thoughts? If yes, are they routine or are they repetitive thoughts that you would rather not have or find disturbing? If yes, are they:)

_____ _____ Forbidden or perverse sexual thoughts, images, impulses

_____ _____ Content involves homosexuality

_____ _____ Sexual behavior towards others (aggressive)

_____ _____ Other (describe): _____

Hoarding/Saving Obsessions

_____ _____ Fear of losing things

_____ _____ Other (describe): _____

Magical Thoughts/Superstitious Obsessions

_____ _____ Lucky/unlucky numbers, colors, words

_____ _____ Other (describe): _____

Somatic Obsessions

_____ _____ Excessive concern with illness or disease

_____ _____ Excessive concern with body part or aspect of appearance (e.g., dysmorphophobia)

_____ _____ Other (describe): _____

Religious Obsessions (Scrupulosity)

_____ _____ Excessive concern or fear of offending religious objects (God)

_____ _____ Excessive concern with right/wrong, morality

_____ _____ Other (describe): _____

Miscellaneous Obsessions

_____ _____ The need to know or remember

_____ _____ Fear of saying certain things

_____ _____ Fear of not saying just the right thing

_____ _____ Intrusive (nonviolent) images

_____ _____ Intrusive sounds, words, music, or numbers

_____ _____ Other (describe): _____

(cont.)

CY-BOCS COMPULSIONS CHECKLIST

Current	Past	

Washing/Cleaning Compulsions

_____ _____ Excessive or ritualized handwashing

_____ _____ Excessive or ritualized showering, bathing, toothbrushing, grooming, toilet routine

_____ _____ Excessive cleaning of items; such as personal clothes or important objects

_____ _____ Other measures to prevent or remove contact with contaminants

_____ _____ Other (describe): _____

Checking Compulsions

_____ _____ Checking locks, toys, school books/items, etc.

_____ _____ Checking associated with getting washed, dressed, or undressed

_____ _____ Checking that did not/will not harm others

_____ _____ Checking that did not/will not harm self

_____ _____ Checking that nothing terrible did/will happen

_____ _____ Checking that did not make mistake

_____ _____ Checking tied to somatic obsessions

_____ _____ Other (describe): _____

Repeating Rituals

_____ _____ Rereading, erasing, or rewriting

_____ _____ Need to repeat routine activities (e.g., in/out of doorway, up/down from chair)

_____ _____ Other (describe): _____

Counting Compulsions

_____ _____ Objects, certain numbers, words, etc.

_____ _____ Describe:

Ordering/Arranging

_____ _____ Need for symmetry/evening up (e.g., lining items up a certain way or arranging personal items in specific patterns)

_____ _____ Other (describe): _____

(cont.)

Hoarding/Saving Compulsions
(distinguish from hobbies and concern with objects of monetary or sentimental value)

_____   _____   Difficulty throwing things away, saving bits of paper, string, etc.

_____   _____   Other (describe): _____

Excessive Games/Superstitious Behaviors
(distinguish from age-appropriate magical games)

_____   _____   (e.g., array of behavior, such as stepping over certain spots on a floor, touching an object/self certain number of times as a routine game to avoid something bad from happening.)

_____   _____   Other (describe): _____

Rituals Involving Other Persons

_____   _____   The need to involve another person (usually a parent) in ritual (e.g., asking a parent to repeatedly answer the same question, making mother perform certain meal-time rituals involving specific utensils).

_____   _____   Other (describe): _____

Miscellaneous Compulsions

_____   _____   Mental rituals (other than checking/counting)

_____   _____   Need to tell, ask, or confess

_____   _____   Measures (not checking) to prevent harm to self ____; harm to others ____; terrible consequences ____

_____   _____   Ritualized eating behaviors

_____   _____   Excessive list making

_____   _____   Need to touch, tap, rub

_____   _____   Need to do things (e.g., touch or arrange) until it *feels* just right

_____   _____   Rituals involving blinking or staring

_____   _____   Trichotillomania (hair-pulling)

_____   _____   Other self-damaging or self-mutilating behaviors

_____   _____   Other (describe): _____

Index

About the Authors

John S. March, MD, is Chief of Child and Adolescent Psychiatry at Duke University Medical Center. Recently, he served as one of the principal investigators of a National Institute of Mental Health–funded project that compared cognitive-behavioral therapy, medication, and a combination of the two for helping kids and teens beat OCD. A widely published author of books for professionals, including *OCD in Children and Adolescents*, his research defines the state of the art for treatment of young people with OCD and other anxiety and mood disorders. In addition to his clinical work, Dr. March is active in the teaching and training of mental health professionals. He lives in Durham, North Carolina.

Christine M. Benton has over 25 years of experience as a writer and editor of books on psychology, self-help, consumer health issues, and other topics. She is coauthor, with Russell A. Barkley, PhD, of *Your Defiant Child: Eight Steps to Better Behavior,* also published by The Guilford Press.